MEL

A Monograph

MELASMA
A Monograph

Editor

Rashmi Sarkar MD MNAMS
Professor
Department of Dermatology
Maulana Azad Medical College and
Associated LNJP Hospital
New Delhi, India

Foreword

Amit G Pandya

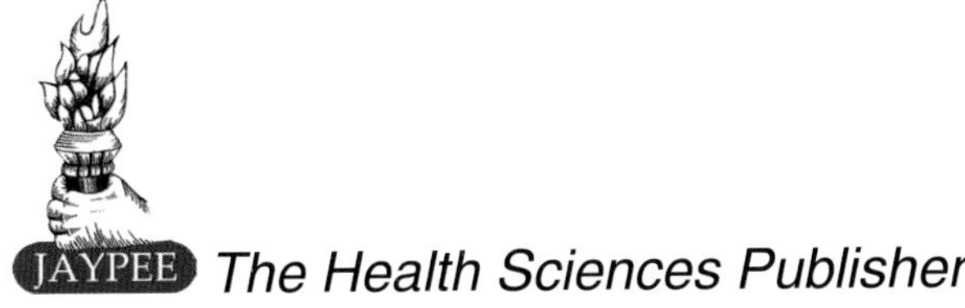

New Delhi | London | Philadelphia | Panama

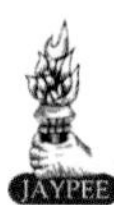

Jaypee Brothers Medical Publishers (P) Ltd

Headquarters

Jaypee Brothers Medical Publishers (P) Ltd
4838/24, Ansari Road, Daryaganj
New Delhi 110 002, India
Phone: +91-11-43574357
Fax: +91-11-43574314
Email: jaypee@jaypeebrothers.com

Overseas Offices

J.P. Medical Ltd
83 Victoria Street, London
SW1H 0HW (UK)
Phone: +44 20 3170 8910
Fax: +44 (0)20 3008 6180
Email: info@jpmedpub.com

Jaypee-Highlights Medical Publishers Inc
City of Knowledge, Bld. 237, Clayton
Panama City, Panama
Phone: +1 507-301-0496
Fax: +1 507-301-0499
Email: cservice@jphmedical.com

Jaypee Medical Inc
The Bourse
111 South Independence Mall East
Suite 835, Philadelphia, PA 19106, USA
Phone: +1 267-519-9789
Email: jpmed.us@gmail.com

Jaypee Brothers Medical Publishers (P) Ltd
17/1-B Babar Road, Block-B, Shaymali
Mohammadpur, Dhaka-1207
Bangladesh
Mobile: +08801912003485
Email: jaypeedhaka@gmail.com

Jaypee Brothers Medical Publishers (P) Ltd
Bhotahity, Kathmandu, Nepal
Phone: +977-9741283608
Email: kathmandu@jaypeebrothers.com

Website: www.jaypeebrothers.com
Website: www.jaypeedigital.com

Inquiries for bulk sales may be solicited at: jaypee@jaypeebrothers.com

Melasma: A Monograph / Rashmi Sarkar

First Edition: **2015**

ISBN: 978-93-5152-543-1

Printed at : Samrat Offset Pvt. Ltd.

Dedicated to

My late father, Dr AK Sarkar,
Two women who stand by me,
My mother, Mrs Chhobi Sarkar and
My mother-in-law, Mrs Bandana Basu
My son, Abhik Sarkar Basu, and
My patients of melasma

Contents

Contributors

Editor

Rashmi Sarkar MD MNAMS
Professor
Department of Dermatology
Maulana Azad Medical College and Associated LNJP Hospital
New Delhi, India

Contributing Authors

Pooja Arora MD DNB MNAMS
Assistant Professor
Department of Dermatology
Dr RML Hospital and PGIMER
New Delhi, India

Shehnaz Z Arsiwala DDV MD
Consultant Dermatologist
Department of Dermatology
Cosmetic Dermatology, and Lasers
Prince Aly Khan Hospital and
Saifee Hospital
Mumbai, Maharashtra, India

Latika Arya MD
Consultant Dermatologist
LA Skin and Aesthetic Clinic and
Dermatology Group
New Delhi, India

Shivani Bansal MD
Senior Resident
Department of Dermatology
Maulana Azad Medical College
New Delhi, India

Joyeeta Chowdhury MD
RMO-Cum-Clinical Tutor
Department of Dermatology
Nil Ratan Sircar Medical College and
Hospital
Kolkata, West Bengal, India

Maria Suzanne L Datuin MD
Consultant
Department of Dermatology
St. Luke's Medical Center Global City
Taguig City, Philippines

Ncoza Dlova MBChB FCDerm
Consultant Dermatologist
Department of Dermatology
Nelson R Mandela School of Medicine
University of KwaZulu-Natal
Durban, South Africa

Shilpa Garg DNB Fellowship in Dermatosurgery
Assistant Professor
Department of Dermatology
Army College of Medical Sciences,
Base Hospital
New Delhi, India

Narendra Gokhale MD
Consultant Dermatologist
Sklinic
31-C, Indrapuri Colony, Bhawarkua
Indore, Madhya Pradesh, India

Evangeline B Handog MD
Chair, Department of Dermatology
Asian Hospital and Medical Center
Consultant and Head
Cosmetic Dermatology Unit
Department of Dermatology
Research Institute for Tropical Medicine
Metro Manila, Philippines

Hee Young Kang MD PhD
Professor
Department of Dermatology
Ajou University School of Medicine
Suwon, Korea

Saloni Katoch MBBS
Final year Post Graduate Trainee
Department of Dermatology
JJM Medical College
Davangere, Karnataka, India

Nokubonga Khoza MBChB FCDerm
Consultant Dermatologist
Department of Dermatology
Nelson R Mandela School of Medicine
University of KwaZulu-Natal
Durban, South Africa

Anisa Mosam MBChB FCDerm MMed PhD
Associate Professor
Department of Dermatology
Nelson R Mandela School of Medicine
University of KwaZulu-Natal
Durban, South Africa

Amit G Pandya MD
Professor
Department of Dermatology
University of Texas Southwestern
Medical Center
Dallas, Texas, USA

Nilendu Sarma MD
Assistant Professor
Department of Dermatology
Nil Ratan Sircar Medical College and
Hospital
Kolkata, West Bengal, India

Sumit Sethi MD
Senior Resident
Department of Dermatology
Maulana Azad Medical College and
Lok Nayak Hospital
New Delhi, India

Sidharth Sonthalia MD MNAMS
Consultant Dermatologist and
Dermatosurgeon
Skinnocence - The Skin Clinic
Gurgaon, Haryana, India

Foreword

The disfiguring stain of melasma is a facial curse affecting millions throughout the world. Although it is not associated with mortality, psychological morbidity may be profound. In this monograph, Dr Rashmi Sarkar and colleagues have produced a succinct and excellent treatise on this disorder, packed with important, up-to-date information. Within a short period of time, physicians can expand their knowledge of melasma exponentially by reading this booklet and apply this information immediately to the next melasma patient who walks through their clinic doors. Virtually, all aspects of this form of dyschromia are covered, including pathogenesis, topical creams, peels, lasers, and impact on quality of life. With recent studies showing the incidence of melasma high in most parts of the world, this publication comes a timely moment for all of us trying to treat patients with this disorder. I commend the contributors and hope you enjoy reading this monograph as much as I did.

Amit G Pandya MD
Professor
Department of Dermatology
University of Texas Southwestern Medical Center
Dallas, Texas, USA

Preface

A monograph on melasma was the first book I had in mind when I thought of writing. However, it stayed in the shelves of my mind quietly, till I co-edited two other books. The idea of completing my pet project came back and with the good wishes of my colleagues who write on this topic, my mentors and my family, I took up editing this book once again. For me this book highlights my area of interest and research over the years and is very close to my heart. I have kept the format simple.

I would like to thank my teachers in PGIMER, Chandigarh, India who always laid special emphasis on "Pigmentary Disorders", my mentors, Dr Amit G Pandya and Dr Pearl E Grimes for making my dreams turn into reality by their encouragement at the American Academy of Dermatology and Dr Vijay Garg, the head of our department for his help and encouragement. A lot has been written on vitiligo but melasma has not received so much attention, hence that was how the idea of writing this "Monograph" was born. A word of thanks to Mr JP Vij at Jaypee Brothers Medical Publishers (P) Ltd. and especially Dr Madhu Choudhary, Ms Shweta Tiwari, and Mr Manoj Kumar who helped in the editorial and designing process and were delightful to work with. A special note of appreciation to Dr Shilpa Garg for helping me in proof reading and editing. Lastly, I appreciate the encouragement from Mr Sathya Narayanan, Mr S Raghavendra, and Mr Sanket Paranjpe and the entire team of Galderma for their belief and support.

A word of thanks to my husband, Dr Srikanta Basu and my son Abhik S Basu for prodding me on always. My patients of melasma and my students remain invaluable to me. As also the various eminent international and national authors, all friends, who came forward to contribute. I hope, you, the reader enjoys reading this book as much as I enjoyed editing and writing it.

Rashmi Sarkar MD MNAMS
Professor
Department of Dermatology
Maulana Azad Medical College and Associated LNJP Hospital
New Delhi, India

CHAPTER 1

Epidemiology and Global Distribution of Melasma

Nokubonga Khoza, Ncoza Dlova, Anisa Mosam

INTRODUCTION

The accurate prevalence of melasma worldwide is unknown. This is attributed to the fact that melasma is a cosmetic problem and most patients may choose to consult their dermatologist privately.[1] Hence, a low prevalence of melasma is recorded in most public dermatology clinics. Unfortunately, these are not truly representative samples.[1,2] According to the American Academy of Dermatology, melasma affects 5–6 million people, mostly women in the United States alone.[2-4]

There have been few studies that have randomly sampled the general population (Table 1).[3]

Although melasma affects all races, it is most prevalent among darker skin phototypes (Fitzpatrick skin III–V) and mainly in patients of Hispanic, Latin Americans, Asian, Middle Eastern, and African descent; these have been the most studied groups (Figure 1).[1-5]

Melasma was noted to be a common cutaneous disorder, accounting for 0.25–4% of patients seen in dermatology clinics in South East Asia and was the most common pigment disorder among Indians. In the Hispanic population in Texas, Werlinger et al. noted the prevalence to be 8.8%, with previous history of melasma in 4% patients.[3,6] In Iraq, melasma is also the most common dermatology problem accounting for 26.6% of Iraqi females. The polarity of melasma towards these ethnic groups is influenced by genetic and environmental

Table 1: Prevalence of melasma

Author	Location	Percentage of cases with melasma
Sivayathorn	Thailand	33%
Sarkar et al.	India	20.5% (in men)
Failmezger	Peru	10.1%
Werliner et al.	USA	8.8%
Tomb and Nassart	Lebanon	3.4%
Parthasaradhi and Al Gufai	Saudi Arabia	2.88%
Hiletework	Ethopia	1.8%

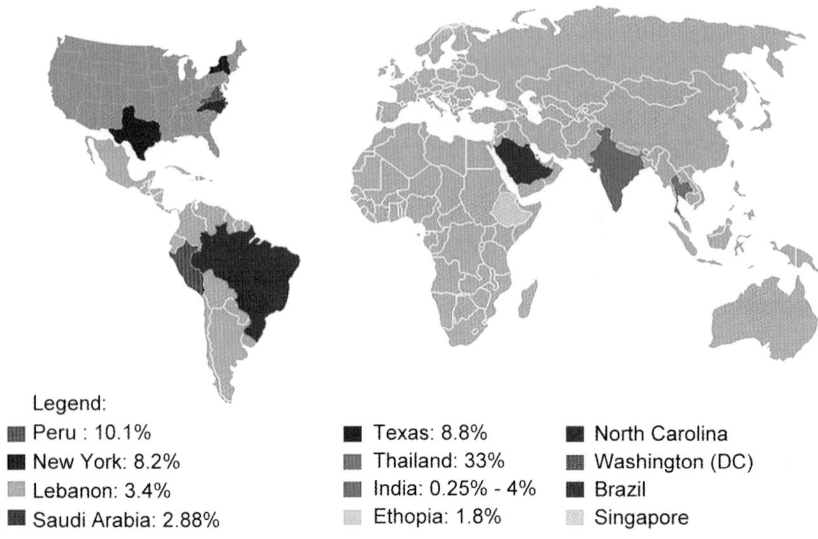

Figure 1: Schematic world map view of reported melasma prevalence and cases.

factors i.e., living in areas of intense ultraviolet light exposure and the fact that physiologically darker skin produces larger amounts of melanin in response to solar radiation.[1]

Hexsel et al. noted that the occurrence of melasma in lighter skin phototypes i.e., Fitzparick skin type II and III was influenced by the presence of family history in contrast to negative family history in Fitzpatrick's phototype IV and V.[7]

Melasma affects women more than men and occurs during child bearing age. The influence on age of onset have been thought to be related to a positive family history; first degree family having greater influence than second degree, and supporting genetic factors in the development of melasma.[2] Krupashankar et al. also concluded that there is a strong correlation between family history and the prevalence of melasma amongst Indian population, this was highlighted by the regional variation in demographics and factors that precipitated melasma in three regions within India.[8] In the Brazilian population, familial melasma is noted, with 50% of patients presenting with melasma having a first degree relative with the disease. In these patients, melasma was associated with long disease duration.[2] Family history was also associated with early age of onset in patients with Fitzpatrick skin type III–V but also in the occurrence of melasma in lighter skin type II.[2,7]

Male melasma is related to excessive ultraviolet light exposure secondarily to occupational and other lifestyle issues in predisposed individuals. Pichardo et al. looking at melasma in immigrant Latino men (poultry processors and manual workers) noted that the prevalence of melasma in Latino men was 14.5% a bit higher than in women.[9] Melasma in these men occurred at a later age of onset 31 years or older. In those whose occupation involved high level of sunlight, presentation occurred at an earlier age.[9] Sarkar et al. also noted a prevalence of melasma to be about 20.5% in men in a prospective study in a tertiary care hospital, New Delhi, India.[10]

The relationship between melasma and pregnancy and hormonal influences in melasma has been documented. Most women with melasma report onset of disease during or after pregnancy or in relation to use of oral contraception. Pregnancy induced melasma is associated with early disease.[2] Few population based studies that have looked at melasma have shown a varying prevalence of 10–70%, suggesting that other factors like ethnicity and sun exposure are significantly involved.[2,4,11]

Although, melasma is a common and easily diagnosed skin condition, better studies are required to address the worldwide epidemiology and prevalence.

Editor's Note

Melasma is definitely among the top five leading dermatologic conditions in Asia. Ethnicity, genetic factors, and sun exposure play important roles. There are hardly any community based studies and global data are mostly based on hospital based studies.

REFERENCES

1. Al-Hamdi KI, Hasony HJ, Jareh HL. Melasma in Basrah: A clinical and Epidemiological study. MJBU. 2008;26:1-5.
2. Tamega AA, Miot LDB, Bonfietti C, Gige TC. Clinical Patterns and Epidemiological characteristics of facial melasma in Brazilian women. J Eur Acad Dermatol. 2013;27:151-6.
3. Sheth VM, Pandya AG. Melasma: A comprehensive update: part I. J Am Acad Dermatol. 2011;65:699-714.
4. Ortonne JP, Arellano I, Berneburg M, Cestari T, Chan H, Grimes P, et al. A global survey of the role of ultraviolet radiation and hormonal influences in the development of melasma. J Eur Acad Dermatol Venereol. 2009;23:1254-62.
5. Achar A, Rathi S. Melasma: A clinico-epidemiological study of 312 cases. Indian J Dermatol. 2011;56:380-2.
6. Werlinger KD, Guevara IL, Gonzalez CM, Rincon ET, Caetano R, Haley RW, et al. Prevalence of self-diagnosed melasma among pre-menopausal Latino women in Dallas and Forth Worth, Tex. Arch Dermatol. 2007;143:424-5.
7. Hexsel D, Lacerda DA, Cavalcante AS, Machado Filho CA, Kalil CL, Ayres EL, et al. Epidemiology of melasma in Brazilian patients: a multicenter study. Int J Dermatol. 2014; 53:440-4.
8. Krupashankar DS, Somani VK, Kohli M, Sharad J, Ganjoo A, Kandhari S. A Cross-Sectional, Multicentric Clinico-Epidemiological Study of Melasma in India. Dermatol Ther (Heidelb). 2014;4:71-81.
9. Pichardo-Geisinger R, Muñoz-Ali D, Arcury TA, Blocker JN, Grzywacz JG, Mora DC, et al. Dermatologist-diagnosed skin diseases among immigrant Latino poultry processors and other manual workers in North Carolina, USA. Int J Dermatol. 2013;52:1342-8.
10. Sarkar R, Puri P, Jain RK, Singh A, Desai A. Melasma in men: a clinical, aetiological and histological study. J Eur Acad Dermatol Venereol. 2010;24:768-72.
11. Dlova NC, Mankahla A, Madala N, Grobler A, TsokaGwegweni J, Hift RJ. The spectrum of skin diseases in a black population in Durban, KwaZuluNatal, South Africa. Int J Dermatol. 2014 (In Press).

CHAPTER 2

Etiological Factors and Triggering Factors

Hee Young Kang

INTRODUCTION

Melasma is a common acquired hyperpigmentary disorder of the sun-exposed area. It is widely accepted that it is more common in women and darker skin types such as Hispanics and Asians. Although the exact prevalence of melasma in general population is unknown, the reported prevalence of melasma ranges from 8.8% among Latino females in the Southern United States to as high as 40% in Southeast Asia.[1] Melasma occurs in 10–15% of pregnant women and 10–25% of women taking oral contraceptives.[2,3] Men represent approximately from about 10% of patients to as high as 20% in Indian melasma patients.[4]

ETIOLOGICAL FACTORS

The major etiological factors include genetic influences, chronic sun exposure, and female sex hormones.[5-8] A large global survey with 324 melasma women confirmed that the combination of the accepted triggering factors do affect onset of melasma.[5] In this study, the mean age at onset of melasma was 34 years (range, 14–65 years) and Fitzpatrick skin phototypes III and IV were most commonly affected. Family history of melasma occurs in about 50% of patients, particularly in patients with darker skin types—African-American. The most common time of onset was after pregnancy (42%) with 26% during pregnancy. Only 25% of patients taking oral contraceptives had an onset of melasma after starting their contraceptive. It was suggested that melasma which first appears during a pregnancy is more likely to resolve spontaneously.[1] The study conclude, that a combination of factors including UV exposure, family history, and hormonal disturbances are likely to play a role in the development of melasma. An epidemiologic study with 302 Brazilian patients with melasma was performed and in these samples, melasma was also common in middle-aged woman with intermediate skin phototypes, Fitzpatrick skin phototypes III and IV.[6] A high familial incidence of more than half the patients was reported and supporting genetic factors are important in developing melasma. It was noted that the patients who had positive family history had longer disease duration. The most commonly reported precipitating factors were pregnancy (36.4%), oral contraceptives (16.2%) and sun exposure (27.2%). It was noted that the pregnancy-associated melasma had earlier onset and was more common in those who had multiple pregnancies. In another multicenter study with 953 Brazilian melasma patients,[7] it was suggested that the age of melasma onset are related to skin phototypes and family history, i.e., Fitzpatrick skin phototypes II and III and positive family history of melasma had early onset of the melasma when compared with skin phototypes IV, V, and VI or absence of family history. The extrafacial melasma was more frequent in postmenopausal women. In an Indian study with 312 cases, a positive family history was observed in 33.3% and about 55.1% of the patients had intense sun exposure.[8] In this study, only 22.4% of the patients reported pregnancy as a triggering or aggravating factor and only 18.4% of them were taking oral contraceptives during their disease process. The study findings suggested that oral contraceptives or even pregnancy may not be a significant contributing factor in developing of melasma.

CONCLUSION

In summary, above studies suggest that sun exposure and/or hormonal stimuli may trigger melasma development in patients who have intrinsic sensitivity to those stimuli. The high incidence of family history in melasma patients suggests that they have a genetic component. The sun exposure and hormonal stimuli are commonly reported triggering factors in those studies. The prolonged sun exposure could stimulate upregulation of certain melanogenic factors in the melasma skin. The presence of local hormones in the skin may play a role in the development of melasma although the exact mechanism is still unclear. It is possible that certain effects induced by sex hormones in the patients are needed additional synergistic events to develop melasma, for example, UV exposure.

Editor's Note

Out of all triggering factors in melasma, sun exposure and hormonal stimuli in a genetically predisposed individual can cause melasma.

REFERENCES

1. Sheth VM, Pandya AG. Melasma: a comprehensive update: part I. J Am Acad Dermatol. 2011;65:689-97.
2. Hexsel D, Rodrigues T, Dal'forno T, Zechmeister-Prado D, Lima M. Melasma and pregnancy in southern Brazil. J Eur Acad Dermatol Venereol. 2008;23:367-8.
3. Moin A, Jabery Z, Fallah N. Prevalence and awareness of melasma during pregnancy. Int J Dermatol. 2006;45:285-8.
4. Sarkar R, Puri P, Jain RK, Singh A, Desai A. Melasma in men: a clinical, aetiological and histological study. J Eur Acad Dermatol Venereol. 2010;24:768-72.
5. Ortonne JP, Arellano I, Berneburg M, Cestari T, Chan H, Grimes P, et al. A global survey of the role of ultraviolet radiation and hormonal influences in the development of melasma. J Eur Acad Dermatol Venereol. 2009;23:1254-62.
6. Tamega AA, Miot LD, Bonfietti C, Gige TC, Marques ME, Miot HA. Clinical patterns and epidemiological characteristics of facial melasma in Brazilian women. J Eur Acad Dermatol Venereol. 2013;27:151-6.
7. Hexsel D, Lacerda DA, Cavalcante AS, Machado Filho CA, Kalil CL, Ayres EL, et al. Epidemiology of melasma in Brazilian patients: a multicenter study. Int J Dermatol. 2014;53:440-4.
8. Achar A, Rathi SK. Melasma: a clinico-epidemiological study of 312 cases. Indian J Dermatol. 2011;56:380-2.

CHAPTER 3

Etiopathogenesis of Melasma

Sidharth Sonthalia

INTRODUCTION

Melasma, one of the most common hyperpigmentary disorders known, is a frustrating condition. Relapse is invariable despite optimum preventive measures and dermatologists can only ensure "treatment and maintenance" of effect rather than "permanent cure". Despite continuous quest for the etiological factors and pathogenetic mechanisms contributing to melasma, its pathophysiology remains elusive and treatment challenging. Over the last one decade, new findings based on advanced techniques like dermoscopy, *in vivo* reflectance confocal microscopy (RCM), and immunohistochemistry from biopsy specimens have provided sufficient insight into its pathogenesis. While old time-tested theories regarding its pathophysiology have not yet been discarded, recent and emerging postulates need further confirmation. Two groups of factors seem to be instrumental: (1) "endogenous factors", most importantly genetic predisposition and cutaneous vasculature and (2) "exogenous stimuli" such as sex hormones and ultraviolet (UV) irradiation, respectively.

EPIDERMAL HYPERPIGMENTATION: THE MAIN CULPRIT

Melasma has traditionally been classified into epidermal, mixed, and dermal. This differentiation by Wood's lamp examination has been *in vogue*, with features of epidermal, dermal, and mixed type of melasma being accentuation of lesional pigmentation, lack of enhancement of lesional pigment, and presence of both enhancing and nonenhancing areas, respectively. However, this concept seems redundant with a recent *in vivo* RCM study that demonstrated heterogenous distribution of melanophages between different regions of the melasma lesion and within a particular region of a melasma lesion. These findings raise serious doubts about the existence of "true epidermal" or "true dermal" melasma and suggest that all melasma are indeed mixed.[1] Epidermal hyperpigmentation through increased melanogenesis in epidermal melanocytes is now considered to be the hallmark of melasma lesional skin, evidenced by an 83% increase in epidermal pigmentation in the lesional skin of 56 Korean patients, and confirmed on RCM.[1,2] Thus, melasma is chiefly characterized by epidermal hyperpigmentation with or without melanophages. The role of small amount of dermal melanin in the melasma lesional skin remains speculative.

MELANOGENESIS, MELANOCYTOSIS, AND HYPERACTIVE MELANOCYTES

Histopathology of melasma lesions has offered valuable insights to understand its etiopathogenesis. In the study by Kang et al. (*vide supra*) comparing the histology of melasma lesions and normal facial skin, the following features were more pronounced in the former—solar elastosis, greater number of epidermal melanocytes, dermal free melanin and melanophages, elastic fiber fragmentation, and significantly increased epidermal melanin.[2] The melanocytes in lesional skin have been found to be biologically more active than their counterparts in normal skin with increased dendriticity and presence of greater quantities of mitochondria, Golgi, and rough endoplasmic reticulum.[3] While enhanced melanogenesis within these melanocytes of melasma lesions has been proven by recent findings of upregulation of many melanin biosynthesis-related genes and melanocytes markers like tyrosinase, TYRP1, TYRP2, and MITF, whether melanocytosis contributes to it is still controversial.[1-3]

MULTIFACTORIAL ETIOPATHOGENESIS OF MELASMA (FIGURE 1)

The major etiological factors implicated in melasma seem to act in concert. In a study of 210 patients, the incidence of different causative factors was: 100% for sunlight exposure, 27% for pregnancy, 14% for cosmetics, 13% for familial factors, and 6.3% for oral contraceptive pill (OCP) use.[4] The results of a recent global survey by Ortonne et al. in 324 women with melasma also suggest that a combination of hormonal factors such as pregnancy and OCP use and sun-exposure are involved.[5]

GENETICS AND RACIAL FACTORS

A genetic predisposition is suggested by a high reported incidence in family members of certain racial groups. It has ranged from 10% to up to 70% in studies from Iran, Singapore, and in Latino men.[6] In Southeast Asia, the prevalence ranged from 40% in females and 20% in males.[7] The global survey by Ortonne et al. comprising of women from nine countries reinforced the susceptibility of Fitzpatrick skin phototypes III and IV and a higher likelihood of a positive family history in African-Americans.[5] The underlying molecular mechanisms need to be elucidated.

ROLE OF SUN EXPOSURE

Facts Suggesting the Relationship of Melasma with Sun Exposure

Sun-exposure, especially UV radiation (UVR) is undoubtedly the most important etiological factor for melasma. Occurrence of lesions in predominantly sun-

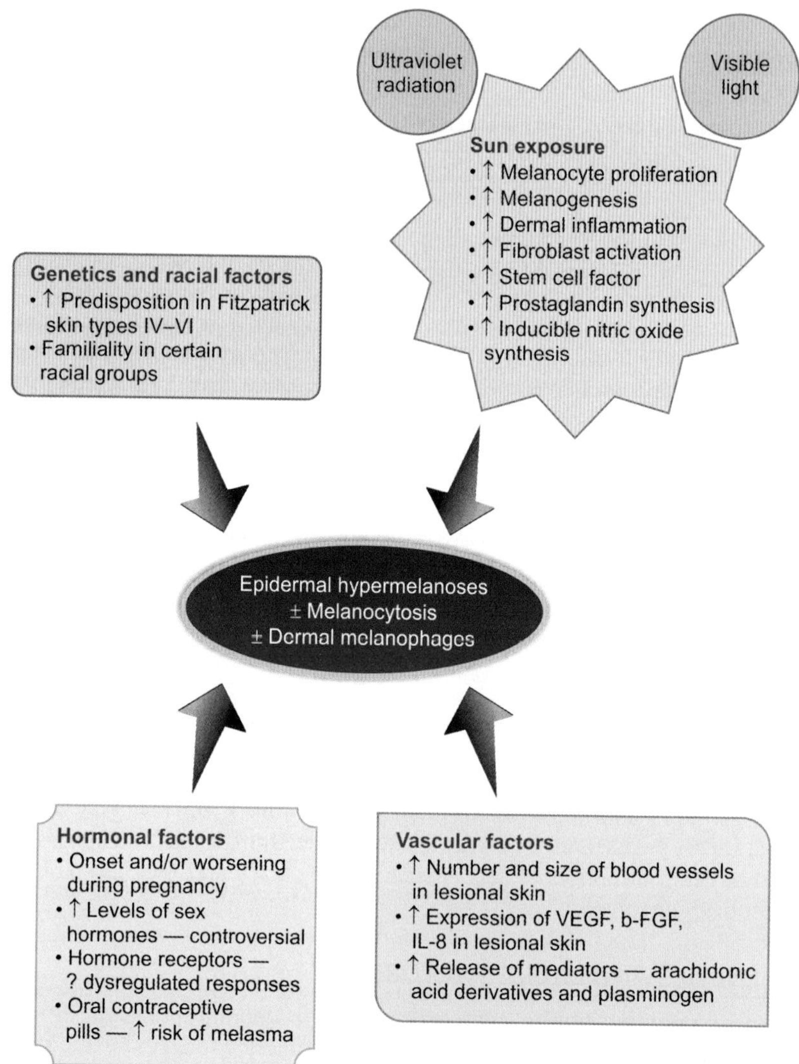

VEGF, vascular endothelial growth factor; b-FGF, basic fibroblast growth factor; IL, interleukin.

Figure 1: Major etiological factors of melasma with mechanisms associated with them.

exposed areas of the face and delay in relapse after successful reduction with regular use of broad-spectrum sunscreens support the role of unimpeded sun-exposure in evolution and progression of melasma. Moreover, features of solar damaged skin, typically solar elastosis on histology, are often present in lesions of melasma.

Cellular and Humoral Mechanisms Underlying UV-induced Melasma

Complex cellular interactions and interplay of cytokines and hormones contribute to the effect of UVR in melasma. Latest evidence has implicated cells other than melanocytes notably, keratinocytes, dermal fibroblasts and cutaneous vasculature.[8]

- *Effects of UVR on keratinocyte-melanocyte interaction*: Melanocyte proliferation, migration, and melanogenesis are upregulated by UVR directly, as well as indirectly by the cytokines like interleukin-1 and endothelin-1, and peptides especially α-melanocyte-stimulating hormone (α-MSH), and adrenocorticotropic hormone (ACTH) produced by UV-stimulated keratinocytes. These peptides stimulate melanocyte proliferation as well as melanin synthesis via stimulation of tyrosinase activity and tyrosinase-related protein 1 (TRP-1).[9] The enhanced expression of inducible nitric oxide synthase (iNOS) in melasma within keratinocytes also contributes to the melanogenesis process[10]
- *Effects of UVR on dermal inflammation and fibroblast activation*: Kang et al. have reported significantly increased expression of both stem cell factor (SCF) from fibroblasts and c-kit in the melasma lesional skin.[11] The cytokines derived from fibroblasts stimulate the proliferation and melanogenesis of melanocytes. Thus, the UV-induced dermal inflammation leading to fibroblast activation resulting in upregulation of SCF in the dermis of melasma lesions, culminating into increased melanogenesis sounds like a plausible explanation. Other inflammatory events operating at the cellular level may also have a role. UV-stimulated synthesis of prostaglandin (PGs) and upregulation of COX2 in lesional skin resulting in epidermal hyperpigmentation has been reported.[2] The emergence of PG analogs as a therapeutic option for vitiligo lends further support to this speculation
- *Visible light and melasma*: Apart from the effect of UVR, the role of visible light is being increasingly recognized. Visible light is known to induce hyperpigmentation especially in skin types IV–VI.[12] It could explain the only partial protective effect of most UV-A and UV-B protective sunscreens and higher efficacy of tinted mineral sunscreens that additionally protect against visible light in prevention of melasma relapses.

It is curious that unlike other photosensitive dermatoses, such as polymorphous light eruption and actinic dermatitis, melasma exclusively involves the face with sparing of other sun-exposed body parts.

ROLE OF HORMONES

The relationship of melasma with female sex hormones, OCPs, and pregnancy has been perplexing and needs further elucidation.

Pregnancy and Melasma

Many patients note the onset or worsening of melasma during pregnancy; often christened as "chloasma gravidarum" and "the mask of pregnancy" with typical onset during the second half of the gestational period. However, melasma may appear before pregnancy or many years after delivery. The reported incidence of melasma appearing during pregnancy has ranged from 2.5% to 75% with genetic and racial factors contributing to this wide variation. Major studies on epidemiology of melasma in Indian women are lacking; however, two studies have reported an incidence of 2.5–8.5% during pregnancy in Indian women.[13,14]

Hormones, Hormone Receptors, and Melasma

Though results of existing studies support the role of a hormonal component in the pathogenesis of melasma, the evidence is not robust due to wide variation in their results owing to the varied genetic backgrounds of different study populations. In the study by Perez et al. comparing basal state serum levels of multiple steroidal and female hormones between nine women with idiopathic melasma (unrelated with pregnancy or OCP intake) and their age- and sex-matched normal controls, the only discernible difference was statistically significant increased levels of luteinizing hormone (LH) and relatively lower levels of serum estradiol in melasma patients.[15] With lack of clarity on the role of levels of circulating levels in pathogenesis of melasma, the role of hormone receptors has become an active area of research. Immunohistochemical studies have shown that compared to melanocytes of non-lesional skin, cells from melasma lesions exhibit increased estrogen receptor expression. However, the response of these receptors to different hormones in melanocyte-incubation studies has also been conflicting with variable changes in melanocyte proliferation and tyrosinase activity. Thus, factors such as heightened sensitivity of melanocytes of melasma lesions to estrogens (and possibly other hormones) and additional synergistic influences such as UVR, cutaneous vasculature, activity of sebaceous glands, and oxidative stress also need to be considered.[6]

Oral Contraceptive Pills and Melasma

The onset of melasma following intake of OCPs is well-documented. In the global survey by Ortonne et al., 25% of 324 women with melasma reported disease onset with OCP use.[5] The accrued evidence from different studies studying the epidemiology of OCP-induced melasma suggests it to be more common in patients lacking family history of melasma and a higher risk of recurrence or worsening of melasma during pregnancy in such patients. Thus, while patients who develop melasma while taking OCPs may benefit by stopping them and avoiding them in future, a systematic change in hormonal contraception in melasma patients seems unwarranted.[5,6]

VASCULAR FACTORS

The demonstration of more prominent solar elastosis in lesional melasma skin compared with perilesional skin, and UV-induced dermal inflammation leading to fibroblast activation and resultant increase in melanogenesis makes a strong case for the role of dermal environment in development of melasma.[2,11] There is a newfangled interest in the role of cutaneous vasculature in its pathogenesis. Though hyperpigmented patches predominate the clinical presentation of melasma, many patients demonstrate additional distinguishing features like pronounced telangiectatic erythema confined to the melasma lesional skin (Figure 2), more evident on dermoscopy (Figure 3). Evidence from recent research including results of colorimetric analysis, immunohistochemical studies, and laser confocal microscopy examination has shown that melasma lesions are more vascularized than the perilesional skin.[6,11] The investigative study conducted by Kim et al. in 50 women with newly-diagnosed melasma has provided robust evidence to support the vascular theory of melasma and probable events involved in it. They demonstrated a significant increase in both

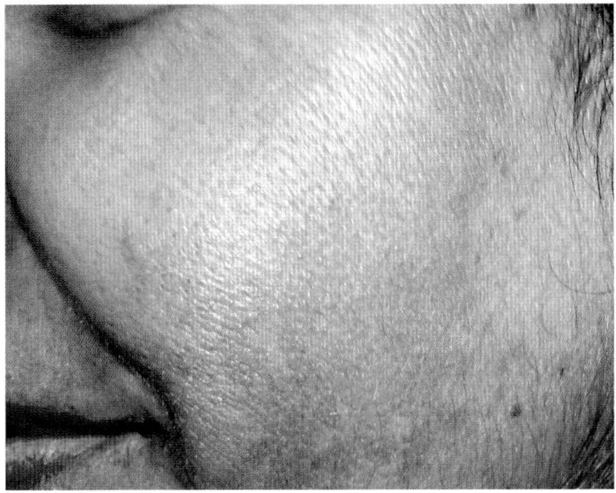

Figure 2: Clinical appearance of an untreated patient with melasma showing pronounced telangiectatic erythema in a background of hyperpigmented macules.

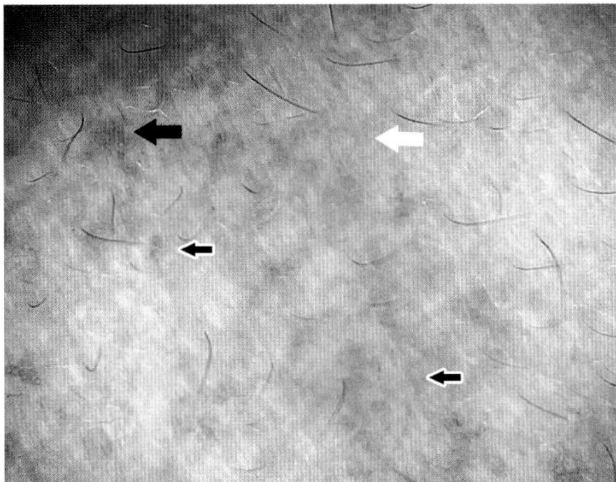

Figure 3: Dermoscopic appearance of the patient in figure 2, demonstrating patchy hyperpigmentation (solid black arrow), prominent interspersed erythema (solid white arrow), and multiple telangiectasias (black arrow with white margins) (original magnification × 10).

the number and size of dermal blood vessels, and upregulated expression of vascular endothelial growth factor (VEGF), in the lesional skin compared to the perilesional normal skin.[16] It has been speculated that UV irradiation induces an angiogenic switch, associated with the upregulation of proangiogenic factors such as VEGF, basic fibroblast growth factor (b-FGF), and interleukin-8. VEGF is the major putative angiogenic factor and it seems to enhance melanogenesis by interaction with VEGF receptors present in epidermal keratinocytes followed by release of mediators, most importantly metabolites of arachidonic acid, and plasminogen from the proliferated vessels.[11,16] The reports of efficacy of two newer treatment modalities, i.e., tranexamic acid, a plasminogen inhibitor, and pulsed dye laser (PDL) that primarily targets vascular components of the skin, further lend support to the vascular theory of melasma.[12]

OTHER FACTORS

Various other factors have been implicated in the pathophysiology of melasma (Table 1). However, the evidence supporting their definitive role is weak and controlled studies are warranted to establish their contribution to the causation of melasma.

Table 1: Minor factors associated with melasma

Causative factor	Association with melasma and possible mechanism
Thyroid disorders	The frequency of thyroid disorders is four times greater in patients with melasma. More commonly associated with hormone-associated melasma
Cosmetics	Photoactive contaminants of mineral oils, petrolatum, beeswax, some dyes, para-phenylenediamine, and perfume ingredients may be involved. While some cases of cosmetic-induced facial hyperpigmentation may actually represent Poikiloderma of Civatte, the role of cosmetic ingredients (in synergism with UV exposure) in causation of melasma cannot be ruled out
Drugs	Phototoxic and photoallergic drugs, e.g., medications containing metals such as arsenic, iron, copper, bismuth, silver, and gold; antiseizure drugs; and organic compounds such as quinacrine have been associated with generalized hyperpigmentation and may be involved with development of melasma
Infection	"*Chlamydia trachomatis*"-induced photosensitivity in patients with clinical or subclinical genitourinary may be contributory, confirmed by the presence of antichlamydia IgM antibodies in many patients with melasma
Stress	Sudden and profound emotional stress implicated in two reports. Release of MSH by the hypothalamus in response to stress is the postulated mechanism
Melanocytic and lentiginous nevi	Patients with melasma tend to show significantly higher number of both types of nevi compared to controls. This indicates a possible relationship between melasma and the overall presence of hyperpigmentary aberrations
Neural component	Increased numbers of keratinocytes expressing nerve growth factor receptor and hypertrophic nerve fibers in the superficial dermis of lesional skin are suggestive of a neural component

UV, ultraviolet; IgM, immunoglobulin M; MSH, melanocyte stimulating hormone.

MOLECULAR PATHOGENESIS

The precise molecular pathogenesis of melasma remains mysterious. Results of a transcriptional analysis study performed in lesional skin samples compared with normal skin have provided interesting insights into its complex pathophysiology. Of the total 279 genes stimulated in this study, 152 were found to be downregulated, with upregulation of many melanogenesis-related genes and melanocytes markers such as TYR, MITF, SILV, and TYRP1.[17] Interestingly, certain genes involved in other biological processes and/or expressed by cells other than melanocytes were found to be differentially expressed in lesional skin, especially a subset of Wnt pathway modulator genes (Wnt inhibitory factor 1, secreted frizzled-related protein 2, and Wnt5a), genes of prostaglandin metabolic processes and those regulating lipid metabolism. Noncoding RNA also seems to participate in the pathogenesis of melasma. In a recent melanocyte–keratinocyte culture study, the H19 gene which transcribes a non-coding RNA was found to be significantly downregulated in lesional skin.[18] Stimulation of melanogenesis and increased transfer of melanin to keratinocytes were associated with decreased transcription of H19 suggesting the role of this gene in evolution of melasma.

Other molecular pathways have also been implicated. Ultraviolet radiation-induced activation of iNOS expression within keratinocytes (*vide supra*) contributing to the melanogenesis process could be linked to an activation of the AKT/NF-κB pathway.[10,12]

CONCLUSION

In summary, though the exact role of etiological factors in causation of melasma and its precise pathogenesis remain puzzling, newer studies have provided corporeal evidence in favor of certain previously suspected and some novel factors. Further research in this area will not only provide more evidence for their involvement in the pathophysiology of melasma, but also offer attractive targets for development of newer treatment modalities.

Editor's Note

Besides the old epidermal-dermal classification of melasma, recent studies show a closer interaction between keratinocytes, melanocytes, and fibrobalasts in pathogenesis of melasma. Vascular factors are also important in the pathogenesis of melasma.

REFERENCES

1. Kang HY, Bahadoran P, Suzuki I, Zugaj D, Khemis A, Passeron T, et al. *In vivo* reflectance confocal microscopy detects pigmentary changes in melasma at a cellular level resolution. Exp Dermatol. 2010;19:228-33.
2. Kang WH, Yoon KH, Lee ES, Kim J, Lee KB, Yim H, et al. Melasma: histopathological characteristics in 56 Korean patients. Br J Dermatol. 2002;146:228-37.
3. Grimes PE, Yamada N, Bhawan J. Light microscopic, immunohistochemical, and ultra-structural alterations in patients with melasma. Am J Dermatopathol. 2005;27:96-101.
4. Katsambas A, Antoniou C. Melasma: Classification and treatment. J Eur Acad Dermatol Venereol. 1995;4:217-23.

5. Ortonne JP, Arellano I, Berneburg M, Cestari T, Chan H, Grimes P, et al. A global survey of the role of ultraviolet radiation and hormonal influences in the development of melasma. J Eur Acad Dermatol Venereol. 2009;23:1254-62.
6. Sheth VM, Pandya AG. Melasma: a comprehensive update: part I. J Am Acad Dermatol. 2011;65:689-97.
7. Sivayathorn A. Melasma in Orientals. Clin Drug Invest. 1995;10:34-40.
8. Kang YH, Ortonne JP. What Should Be Considered in Treatment of Melasma. Ann Dermatol. 2010;22:373-8.
9. Suzuki I, Kato T, Motokawa T, Tomita Y, Nakamura E, Katagiri T. Increase of pro-opiomelanocortin mRNA prior to tyrosinase, tyrosinase-related protein 1, dopachrome tautomerase, Pmel-17/gp100, and P-protein mRNA in human skin after ultraviolet B irradiation. J Invest Dermatol. 2002;118:73-8.
10. Jo HY, Kim CK, Suh IB, Ryu SW, Ha KS, Kwon YG, et al. Co-localization of inducible nitric oxide synthase and phosphorylated Akt in the lesional skins of patients with melasma. J Dermatol. 2009;36:10-6.
11. Kang HY, Hwang JS, Lee JY, Ahn JH, Kim JY, Lee ES, et al. The dermal stem cell factor and c-kit are overexpressed in melasma. Br J Dermatol. 2006;154:1094-9.
12. Passeron T. Melasma pathogenesis and influencing factors—an overview of the latest research. J Eur Acad Dermatol Venereol. 2013;27:5-6.
13. Raj S, Khopkar U, Kapasi A, Wadhwa SL. Skin in pregnancy. Indian J Dermatol Venereol Leprol. 1992;58:84-8.
14. Kumari R, Jaisankar TJ, Thappa DM. A clinical study of skin changes in pregnancy. Indian J Dermatol Venereol Leprol. 2002;73:141.
15. Perez M, Sanchez JL, Aguilo F. Endocrinologic profile of patients with idiopathic melasma. J Invest Dermatol. 1983;81:543-5.
16. Kim EH, Kim YC, Lee ES, Kang HY. The vascular characteristics of melasma. J Dermatol Sci. 2007;46:111-6.
17. Kang HY, Suzuki I, Lee DJ, Ha J, Reiniche P, Aubert J, et al. Transcriptional profiling shows altered expression of wnt pathway- and lipid metabolism-related genes as well as melanogenesis-related genes in melasma. J Invest Dermatol. 2011;131:1692-700.
18. Kim NH, Lee CH, Lee AY. H19 RNA downregulation stimulated melanogenesis in melasma. Pigment cell Melanoma Res. 2010;23:84-92.

CHAPTER 4

Clinical Features and Classification of Melasma, Wood's Lamp, and Melasma Area Severity Index Score

Nilendu Sarma, Joyeeta Chowdhury

INTRODUCTION

Melasma is a common, acquired hypermelanosis that occurs in sun-exposed areas, mostly on the face, occasionally on the neck, and rarely on the forearms. This is resistant to treatment and often causes significant psychological impact on the patient.

It is derived from the Greek word "melas" meaning black. The term, "chloasma" (from the Greek word, "chloazein" meaning "to be green"), is often used to describe melasma developing during pregnancy.[1]

Melasma is a very common cutaneous disorder. The disease affects all races, but there is a particular prominence among Hispanics and Asians.

This is seen in 0.25–4% of the patients in South East Asia, and is possibly the most common pigment disorder among Indians.[2,3] People with darker skin type (Fitzpatrick type IV, V, and VI) are more prone to develop melasma.

It affects all races and sex. However, this is more commonly seen in females. The reported prevalence of melasma in Southeast Asia is 40% of females and 20% of males.[3]

ETIOLOGY

The exact causes of melasma are unknown and are known to be complex. Genetic predisposition is suggested with at least one-third of patients reporting other family members to be affected. Factors known to induce or aggravate melasma are discussed below.

Sun Exposure

This is the most important avoidable risk factor. Distribution of melasma exclusively over the sun-exposed areas and frequent exacerbation of melasma following prolonged sun exposure are supporting evidence.

Melanocyte proliferation, migration and melanogenesis are induced by ultraviolet (UV) rays. Additionally, UV rays stimulates different cytokines like interleukin-1, endothelin-1, α-melanocyte-stimulating hormone (α-MSH), and adrenocorticotropic hormone (ACTH) from keratinocytes. These potentiate melanogenesis.

Pregnancy

It is known to provoke melasma. In a survey, about 41% of women[4] suffering from melasma developed this after pregnancy but before menopause. Pigment getting faded few months after delivery is also reported. However, spontaneous remission might have been over-reported in the past. In a recent study, this may not be seen in only 8% of the cases.

Hormone

Hormone therapy in the form of oral contraceptive pills containing estrogen and/or progesterone, hormone replacement, intrauterine devices, and implants are reported to induce/aggravate melasma in about a quarter of affected women.

Cosmetics

Cosmetics, especially the perfumed ones and soaps may cause a phototoxic reaction triggering melasma that may then persist long-term.[6,7]

Phototoxic Topical Agents

Melasma may develop as phototoxic reaction to certain medications.

Melasma has been found to have higher prevalence of hypothyroidism. The implication of this finding is yet to be elucidated.

CLINICAL APPEARANCE

The hyperpigmented light to dark brown or muddy brown patches develop slowly and may range from single to multiple, usually symmetrical on the face and occasionally on the V-neck area.

According to the distribution of lesions, three clinical patterns of melasma are recognized.[5]

1. The "centrofacial pattern" is the most common pattern (affecting 63% of all cases) and involves the forehead, cheeks, upper lip, nose, and chin (Figure 1).

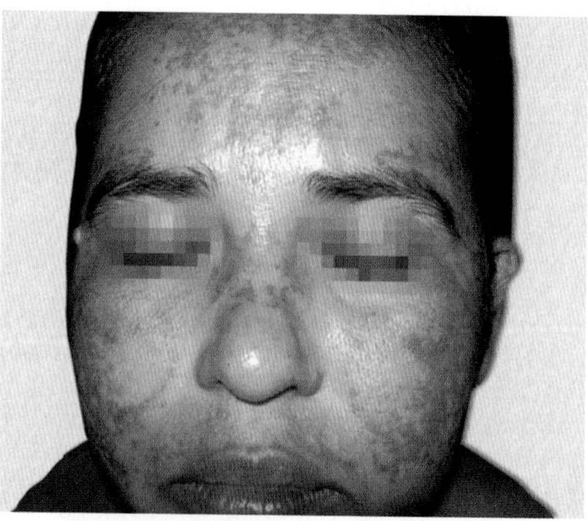

Figure 1: Patient showing brownish non-homogenous pigmented patches over forehead, nose, malar areas, and upper lip.

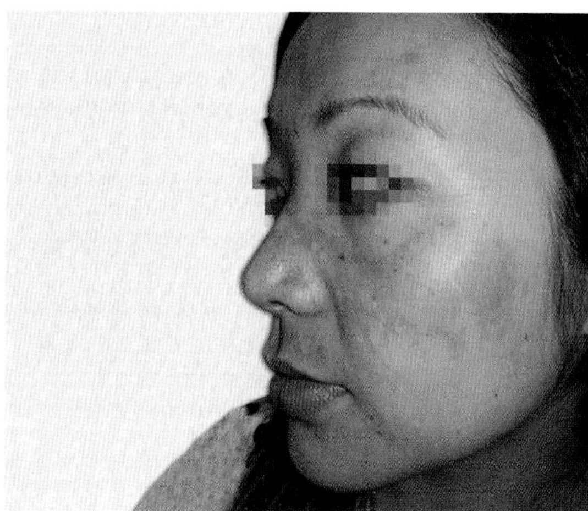

Figure 2: Patient showing diffuse brownish pigmented patches over malar areas and nose.

2. The "malar pattern"(21%) involves the cheeks and nose (Figure 2).
3. The "mandibular pattern"(16%) involves the ramus of the mandible.

DEPTH OF PIGMENTATION

Using the Wood's light examination, melasma can be classified into four major histological types depending upon the depth of pigment deposition.

Epidermal Type

Pigmentation is intensified under Wood's light and is the most common type. Melanin is increased in all epidermal layers.

Dermal Type

Pigmentation is not intensified under Wood's light. It has many melanophages throughout the entire dermis.

Mixed Type

Presence of both the epidermal and dermal patterns noted.

Indeterminate

In dark skinned patients, there is a fourth type, indeterminate, as it may not be discernible in dark skin and minimally contributory.

Recent understanding based on histologic or electron microscopic studies suggest that clear cut distinction in such grouping may not be accurate.

Clinically, the epidermal type is known to have well-defined border, more brown tone, and its response to treatment is much better in comparison to deeper variants. On the other hand, dermal type has ill-defined border.

DIFFERENTIAL DIAGNOSIS

Several conditions may come into the differential diagnosis of melasma like acquired idiopathic facial pigmentation (zygomatic pigmentation/pigmentary demarcation lines),[8] postinflammatory hyperpigmentation, actinic lichen planus, facial acanthosis nigricans, frictional melanosis, acquired bilateral nevus of Ota-like macules (Hori's nevus), nevus of Ota- and drug-induced pigmentation. Early lesions of melasma appear as small macules and often appear as solar lentigines andephelides.

MASI SCORING

Melasma area severity index (MASI) score is calculated with the following formula:[9]

Forehead 0.3 (D + H)A + right malar 0.3 (D + H)A + left malar 0.3 (D + H)A + chin 0.1 (D + H)A.

The severity of the melasma in each of the four regions (forehead, right malar region, left malar region and chin) is assessed based on three variables: (1) percentage of the total area involved (A), (2) darkness (D), and (3) homogeneity (H).

A numerical value assigned for the corresponding percentage of area involved is as follows: 0 = no involvement; ≥1 = 10% involvement; 2 = 10–29% involvement; 3 = 30–49% involvement; 4 = 50–69% involvement; 5 = 70–89% involvement, and 6 = 90–100% involvement.

The darkness of the melasma (D) is compared to the normal skin and graded on a scale of 0–4 as follows: 0 = normal skin color without evidence of hyperpigmentation; 1 = barely visible hyperpigmentation; 2 = mild hyperpigmentation; 3 = moderate hyperpigmentation, and 4 = severe hyperpigmentation.

Homogeneity of the hyperpigmentation (H) is also graded on a scale of 0–4 as follows: 0 = normal skin color without evidence of hyperpigmentation; 1 = specks of involvement; 2 = small patchy areas of involvement less than 1.5 cm diameter; 3 = patches of involvement greater than 2 cm diameter; and 4 = uniform skin involvement without any clear areas).

To calculate the MASI score, the sum of the severity grade for darkness (D) and homogeneity (H) is multiplied by the numerical value of the areas (A) involved and by the percentages of the four facial areas (10–30%). The range of scores is 0–48.

MODIFIED MASI SCORING

Recently, a modified MASI scoring by Pandya et al. was observed to be a reliable scale for measurement of melasma severity.[10] It was seen that only area of involvement and darkness were sufficient for measuring melasma severity. Homogenity was eliminated and the range of scores were from 0–24. The modified MASI score appeared easier to perform.

Modified MASI total score = 0.3 A(f) D(F) + 0:3 A(lm)D(lm) + 0.3 A(rm) D(rm) + 0.1A(c)D(c)

Area and darkness are scored as follows. A area of involvement: 0 = absent, 1 = <10%, 2 = 10%–29%, 3 = 30%–49%, 4 = 50%–69%, 5 = 70%–89%, and 6 = 90%–100%; darkness: 0 = absent, 1 = slight, 2 = mild, 3 = marked, and 4 = severe.

Editor's Note

Wood's lamp examination is a cheap but not very effective investigative tool for classifying melasma. However, it is easy to perform. Melasma area severity index is a subjective scoring system, as many other investigative tools are not easily available everywhere.

REFERENCES

1. Bandyopadhyay D. Topical treatment of melasma. Indian J Dermatol. 2009;54:303-9.
2. Pasricha JS, Khaitan BK, Dash S. Pigmentary disorders in India. Dermatol Clin. 2007;25: 343-52.
3. Sivayathorn A. Melasma in Orientals. Clin Drug Investig. 1995;10:24-40.
4. Ortonne JP, Arellano I, Berneburg M, Cestari T, Chan H, Grimes P, et al. A global survey of the role of ultraviolet radiation and hormonal influences in the development of melasma. J Eur Acad Dermatol Venereol. 2009;23:1254-62.
5. Mosher DB, Fitzpartick TB, Ortonne JP. Hypomelanoses and hypermelanoses. In: Freedburg IM, Eisen AZ, Woeff K, editors. Dermatology in general medicine. 5th ed. New York: McGraw-Hill; 1999. pp. 945-1016.
6. Grimes PE. Melasma: etiologic and therapeutic considerations. Arch Dermatol. 1995;131: 1453-7.
7. Achar A, Rathi SK. Melasma:A clinic-epidemiological study of 312 cases. Indian J Dermatol. 2011;56:380-2.
8. Sarma N, Chakraborty S, Bhattacharya SR. Acquired, idiopathic, patterned facial pigmentation (AIPFP) including periorbital pigmentation and pigmentary demarcation lines on face follows the Lines of Blaschko on face. Indian J Dermatol. 2014;59:41-8.
9. Kimbrough-Green CK, Griffiths CE, Finkel LJ, Hamilton TA, Bulengo-Ransby SM, Ellis CN, et al. Topical retinoic acid (tretinoin) for melasma in black patients. A vehicle-controlled clinical trial. Arch Dermatol. 1994;130:727-33.
10. Pandya AG, Hynan LS, Bhore R,et al. Reliability assessment and validity of the Melasma Area and Severity Index(MASI) and a new modified MASI scoring method. J Am Acad Dermatol 2011;78:78-83.

CHAPTER 5

Investigations in Melasma: Histopathology, Dermoscopy, and *In Vivo* Reflectance Confocal Microscopy in Melasma

Hee Young Kang

HISTOPATHOLOGY

Pigmentation

Histological examinations of melasma have consistently shown that lesional skin is characterized by an increased melanin deposition in the all layers of the epidermis (Figure 1).[1,2] There was an 83% increase in epidermal pigmentation in lesional skin of 56 Korean melasma patients.[1] Another study showed a 61% increase in epidermal pigmentation in lesional skin in all 11 melasma patients of Fitzpatrick skin type IV to VI.[2] The findings have suggested that there is no true

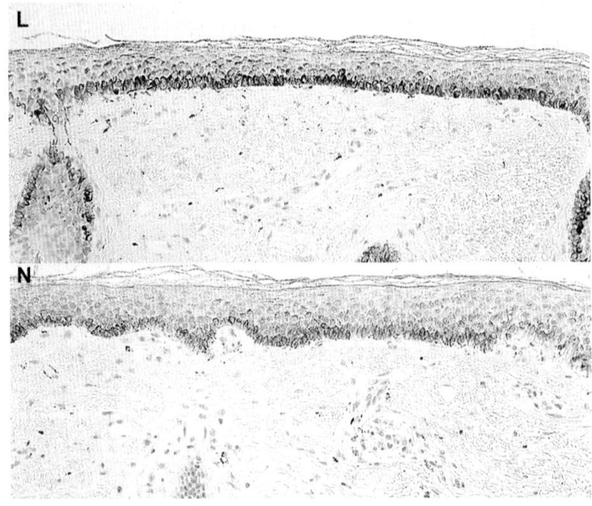

Figure 1: Increased epidermal pigmentation in melasma. Fontana-Masson staining shows more pronounced epidermal hyperpigmentation in lesion (L) compared to perilesional normal skin (N). It is noticed that there are a few melanophages in the dermis of the lesional skin (L) and also in the perilesional normal skin (N).

dermal type of melasma.[1,2] Melanophages were present both in melasma lesional and perilesional normal skin in 36% of Korean patients and in all the melasma patients of Fitzpatrick skin type IV to VI.[1,2] There was no statistically significant difference in the amount of dermal melanin in lesional skin compared to that of perilesional normal skin, although there was slight increase in the lesion.[1,2] The dermal melanophages are commonly found in the sun-exposed skin and the normal facial skin has pigments in the dermis. Therefore, regarding the pigmentation level, melasma is characterized by epidermal hyperpigmentation with or without melanophages.

Melanocytes

The number of melanocytes in melasma is normal or slightly increased. NKI/beteb immunostaining showed an increase in the number of melanocytes, while Mel-5 or MITF staining did not confirm this finding.[1,2] The melanocytes within the lesional skin are larger, intensely stained with prominent dendrites and contain more melanosomes, suggesting that the cells are active. There was upregulation of many melanogenesis-related genes such as tyrosinase, TYRP1, TYRP2, and MITF in lesional skin compared to perilesional normal skin. An interesting feature observed on histopathology is the melanocytes showing a feature of protruding into the dermis, so called pendulous melanocytes.[3-5] The protruding cells were observed in half of melasma specimens.[3] These cells hung down from the basement membrane and was suggested that the loosening of basement membrane is related to the pendulous change of the melanocytes.[4,5] On the reflectance confocal microscopy (RCM) images, these cells appeared as dendritic cells, in which the morphology suggests hyperactivity of the cells.[6] However, the pendulous melanocytes are not pathognomonic for melasma and also observed in other hyperpigmentary disorders, such as solar lentigines and even in normal black skin.

Basement Membrane

The basement membrane structure in melasma lesional skin is not intact and looks disrupted.[4,5] The overall type IV collagen expression was significantly reduced in lesional skin compared with perilesional normal skin.[4] The feature was more evident at the margin of pendulous melanocytes. It was suggested that chronic UV irradiation is responsible for the loosening of basement membrane through upregulation of MMP2 expression in melasma.[4] The change in the basement membrane was suggested to be related to facilitate the interaction between factors secreted from the dermis and epidermal melanocytes to develop melasma.

Dermal Changes

Melasma has alteration in dermal structures in addition to pigmentation changes, suggesting role of dermis for melasma development.[6-8] Increased solar elastosis in lesional skin and increased mast cells localized to elastotic area in melasma have been shown.[6] Overexpression of both stem cell factor (SCF) from fibroblast and increased number of fibroblast have been found in melasma.[7] Melasma lesions have more vascularization as compared to the perilesional normal skin.[8]

The number of vessels had a positive relationship with epidermal pigmentation in melasma lesional skin. Increased expression of vascular endothelial growth factor (VEGF) in keratinocytes was suggested as the major angiogenic factor for altered vessels in melasma. The all findings have suggested that during sun exposure, network of cellular interactions between keratinocytes, fibroblasts, and perhaps vasculature and melanocytes may play an important role in the development of epidermal hyperpigmentation in melasma.

DERMOSCOPY AND *IN VIVO* REFLECTANCE CONFOCAL MICROSCOPY

Dermoscopic examination of melasma revealed irregular pigmentation with a fine brown reticular pattern and capillary vessels in some parts of the lesions. *In vivo* RCM images of melasma showed characteristic significantly increased hyper-refractile cobblestone pattern at the level of basal cell layer in lesional skin compared with perilesional normal skin supporting the existence of epidermal hyperpigmentation in all melasma lesional skin (Figure 2A).[5] Melanophages were recognized in melasma skin in as much as 34.5% of patients and also in the control adjacent skin of four of these patients but to a lesser extent. Most melasma skin showed an abrupt transition from stratum spinosum to papillary dermis and moderately refractile lacy structures (solar elastosis) in the dermis, suggesting the existence of chronic solar damage in the melasma. The all findings are in agreement with available reports regarding histological changes in melasma. A new finding through noninvasive property of RCM is that the distribution of melanophages in melasma is not homogeneous.[5] The distribution of melanophages is very heterogeneous because it can vary from one melasma region to another and even inside a given melasma region.

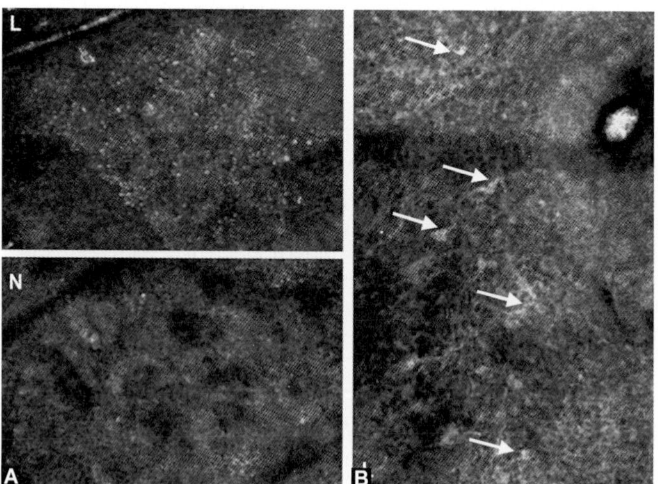

Figure 2: Reflectance confocal microscopy images of melasma. **A,** Increased cobblestonings and loss of dermal papillary rings at the basal layer in lesion (L) compared to perilesional normal skin (N); **B,** Dendritic cells (arrowheads) at the level of dermoepidermal junction of the lesional skin (L).

Another new finding of RCM images of melasma is detected hyperactivated melanocytes in some patients (6/25 patients) of melasma (Figure 2B).[5] On the RCM images, the cells were shown as bright dendritic cells at the level of the dermoepidermal junction in melasma. Immunohistochemical studies confirmed that these cells corresponded to melanocytes, not Langerhans cells. Interestingly, recent study has suggested that the cases showing the presence of these dendritic cells had an early relapse of melasma after treatment.[9] It was also shown that the pigmentary lesion of melasma is rather heterogeneous and in heavily pigmented areas, the dendrites of melanocytes are frequently observed around the basal layer.[10]

The noninvasive nature of this technique suggests that RCM is a suitable tool for treatment monitoring.[9,11] In parallel to the clinical improvement, it was noted a statistically significant decrease in pigmented cells on RCM images after treatment.[11] Interestingly, the cases showing the presence of dendritic cells had an early relapse of melasma after laser toning treatment.[9] This clinical outcome further supported the hypothesis that these cells correspond to activated melanocytes and open the question whether the laser treatment should be stopped or differently modulated in these cases.

Editor's Note

Reflectance confocal microscopy is a noninvasive investigation for melasma and is suitable for monitoring the treatment as opposed to histopathology and dermoscopy alone.

REFERENCES

1. Kang WH, Yoon KH, Lee ES, Kim J, Lee KB, Yim H, et al. Melasma: histopathological characteristics in 56 Korean patients. Br J Dermatol. 2002;146:228-37.
2. Grimes PE, Yamada N, Bhawan J. Light microscopic, immunohistochemical, and ultrastructural alterations in patients with melasma. Am J Dermatopathol. 2005;27:96-101.
3. Lee DJ, Park KC, Ortonne JP, Kang HY. Pendulous melanocytes: a characteristic feature of melasma and how it may occur. Br J Dermatol. 2012;166:684-6.
4. Torres-Álvarez B, Mesa-Garza IG, Castanedo-Cázares JP, Fuentes-Ahumada C, Oros-Ovalle C, Navarrete-Solis J, et al. Histochemical and immunohistochemical study in melasma: evidence of damage in the basal membrane. Am J Dermatopathol. 2011;33:291-5.
5. Kang HY, Bahadoran P, Suzuki I, Zugaj D, Khemis A, Passeron T, et al. *In vivo* reflectance confocal microscopy detects pigmentary changes in melasma at a cellular level resolution. Exp Dermatol. 2010;19:e228-33.
6. Hernández-Barrera R, Torres-Alvarez B, Castanedo-Cazares JP, Oros-Ovalle C, Moncada B. Solar elastosis and presence of mast cells as key features in the pathogenesis of melasma. Clin Exp Dermatol. 2008;33:305-8.
7. Kang HY, Hwang JS, Lee JY, Ahn JH, Kim JY, Lee ES, et al. The dermal stem cell factor and c-kit are overexpressed in melasma. Br J Dermatol. 2006;154:1094-9.
8. Kim EH, Kim YC, Lee ES, Kang HY. The vascular characteristics of melasma. J Dermatol Sci. 2007;46:111-6.
9. Longo C, Pellacani G, Tourlaki A, Galimberti M, Bencini PL. Melasma and low-energy Q-switched laser: treatment assessment by means of in vivo confocal microscopy. Lasers Med Sci. 2014;29:1159-63.
10. Funasaka Y, Mayumi N, Asayama S, Takayama R, Kosaka M, Kato T, et al. In vivo reflectance confocal microscopy for skin imaging in melasma. J Nippon Med Sch. 2013;80:172-3.
11. Tsilika K, Levy JL, Kang HY, Duteil L, Khemis A, Hughes R, et al. A pilot study using reflectance confocal microscopy (RCM) in the assessment of a novel formulation for the treatment of melasma. J Drugs Dermatol. 2011;10:1260-4.

CHAPTER 6

Investigations in Melasma: Dermoscopy in Melasma

Saloni Katoch

INTRODUCTION

Melasma is a common acquired hyperpigmentary disorder occurring mainly on sun-exposed skin on the face and is often a cause for social stigma and embarrassment. Dermoscopy in melasma is an evolving domain, some dermoscopic patterns being consistent with this disorder thereby aiding in its diagnosis and therapeutic monitoring.

On dermoscopic examination of melasma the following can be appreciated:

- *Pattern*: Reticular pattern is the global feature seen in all melasma lesions. This can be superimposed by blotches, globules, and granules. Sparing of sweat gland and follicular openings produce the pseudonetwork pattern with concave borders referred to as the "jelly sign"[1] (Figure 1)
- *Color*: The color of melanin is observed accurately depending upon the amount of pigment, depth and location; going from black when localized in the stratum corneum, shades of brown in the lower layers, to blue or bluish-gray in the dermis[2] (Figures 2 and 3)

Figure 1: Reticuloglobular brown pigmentation (epidermal melasma).

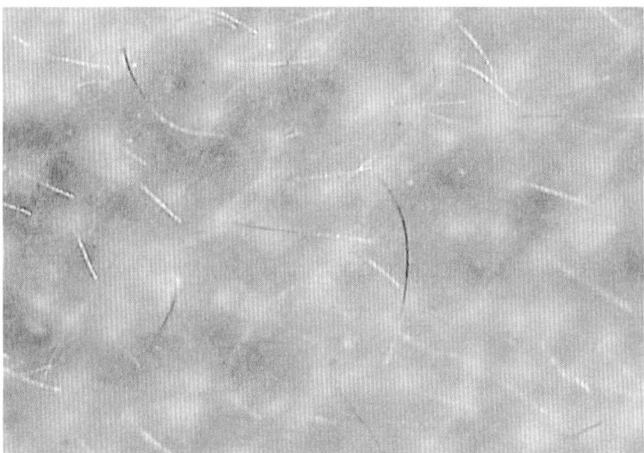

Figure 2: Blue-gray pigmentation (dermal melasma).

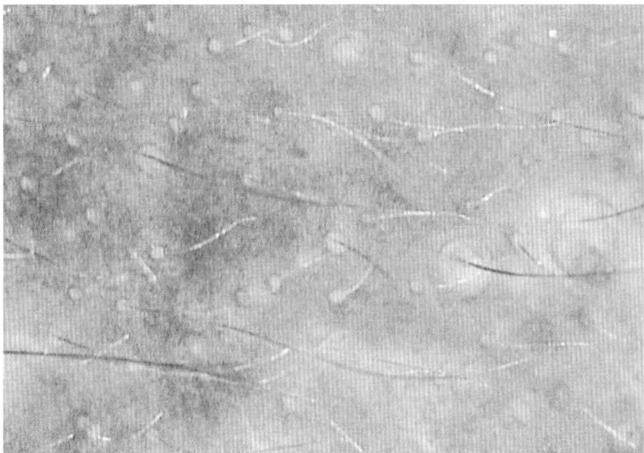

Figure 3: Gray-brown pigmentation (mixed melasma).

- *Others*: Dermoscopy can aid in detecting complications arising due to topical medications like atrophy, telangiectasia, depigmentation, exogenous ochronosis, and steroid dermatitis (Figures 4 and 5).

In a comparative study between dermoscopy and Wood's lamp in classification of melasma, the authors considered the former applicable, more appropriate, and helpful for routine diagnosis, assessment, and monitoring of patients with melasma. Dermoscopic examination allows an objective classification of melasma based on the color of pigment observed. Epidermal type being brownish with a regular pigmented network; dermal type with shades of bluish-gray, the network losing regularity; and the mixed type with features compatible with both.[2]

Dermoscopic evaluation is important for an improved diagnosis of the melasma type, differentiating it from other facial hyperpigmentary conditions, prognosis, and for monitoring treatment efficacy with a potential to detect complications thereby improving the management of our patients.

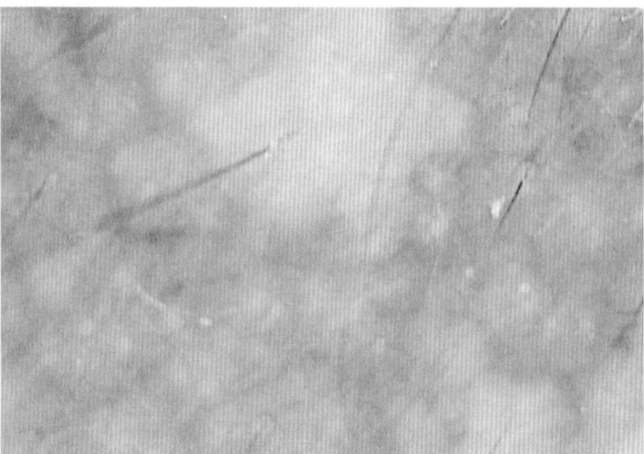

Figure 4: Post-treatment depigmentation.

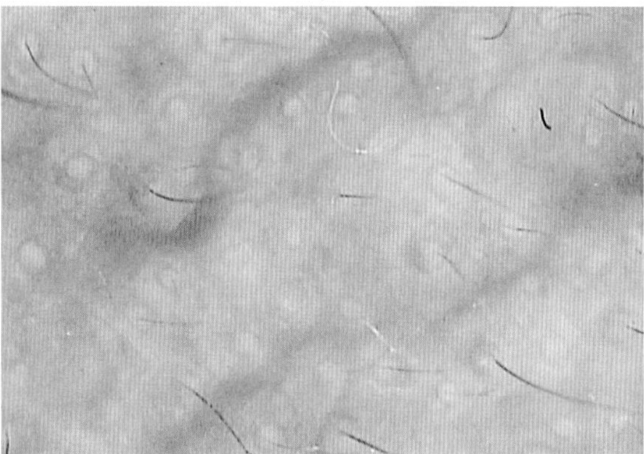

Figure 5: Telangiectasia with areas of pigment clearance.

Acknowledgement

I would like to thank Dr SB Murugesh (Professor and Head, Department of Dermatology, Venereology and Leprology, JJM Medical College, Davangere) for his constant support and guidance.

Editor's Note

Dermoscopy is an evolving science and may help to pick up epidermal, dermal, and mixed melasma as well as various complications of treatment. It is one more useful tool available to the dermatologist.

REFERENCES

1. Mahajan SA. Melasma. In: Khopkar U, editor. Dermoscopy and trichoscopy in diseases of the brown skin. New Delhi: Jaypee Brothers Medical Publishers (P) Ltd.; 2012. pp. 50-62.
2. Talmer C, Fonseca RMR, Pereira FBC, Barcaui CB. Classification of melasma by dermoscopy: comparative study with Wood's lamp. Surg Cosmetic Dermatol. 2009;1:115-9.

CHAPTER 7

Photoprotection and Cosmetic Camouflage for Melasma

Narendra Gokhale

ELECTROMAGNETIC RADIATION

The energy from the sun reaches to us as electromagnetic waves[1] (Table 1).

Table 1: Spectrum of electromagnetic radiation

Wave-length	200–290 nm	290–320 nm	320–340 nm	340–400 nm	400–700 nm	>700 nm
Name	UVC	UVB	UVA2	UVA1	Visible	Infrared

UVA, ultraviolet A; UVB, ultraviolet B; UVC, ultraviolet C.

Pigmentation following Ultraviolet Exposure

Pigment production occurs in skin following both ultraviolet A (UVA) and ultraviolet B (UVB) exposure (Tables 2 and 3).

Ultraviolet A induces three types of pigmentation:

1. Immediate pigment darkening (IPD) develops rapidly in minutes and it also fades rapidly.

Table 2: Effect of different ultraviolet wavelengths on skin[2-4]

Type	UVB	UVA
Effect	• Absorbed by DNA and proteins • Direct damage • Sunburn • Cancer	• Not absorbed by DNA • Penetrates deeper • Aging • Tanning • Immunosuppression • Photocarcinogenesis • Exogenous photodermatitis • Idiopathic photodermatoses

UVA, ultraviolet A; UVB, ultraviolet B; DNA, deoxyribonucleic acid.

Table 3: Time-dependent effects of ultraviolet radiation on skin	
Immediate	**Delayed**
Sunburn UVB	Tanning UVA
Tanning UVB	Aging UVA
Vitamin D synthesis	Malignancy UVB
Thickening	Immunological changes

UVA, ultraviolet A; UVB, ultraviolet B.

2. Persistent pigment darkening (PPD) develops in few hours and may persist for many weeks depending on the UVA dose and the skin type.
3. Delayed pigmentation starts after some days and is long lasting. It is due to increased melanin synthesis.[4]

Ultraviolet B induced tanning is a delayed pigmentation due to melanin synthesis, usually following a burn, and disappears with epidermal turnover.

In darker skinned individuals, UVA has greater pigmenting effects than UVB.

PHOTOPROTECTION

Box 1: General measures[3]

- Avoid sun throughout the day
- Wear broad hats, scarves, dupattas whenever going out
- Keep to the shade when outside
- Avoid scented cosmetics and wet wipes

SUNSCREENS

Sunscreens are over the counter drugs which are applied with the intention to prevent sunlight from reaching the skin[2,3,5-7] (Table 4). Words such as sunblock are not acceptable.

Table 4: The ideal sunscreen
Broad spectrum (covers UVB + UVA2 + UVA1)
Photostable
Good substantivity
Cosmetically acceptable
Water resistant
Nonsensitizing
Fragrance free
Cost effective

UVA, ultraviolet A; UVB, ultraviolet B.

Classification of Ingredients

Sunscreens are divided into organic and inorganic depending on the mechanism of action. The terms physical and chemical are no longer used. There are three commonly used nomenclatures for sunscreen agents in the world. These are the International Nomenclature Cosmetic Ingredient (INCI) name, United States Adopted Name (USAN), and trade name.[8]

Inorganic Sunscreens

These inorganic sunscreens reflect and scatter UV radiation. Inorganic sunscreens are excellent for heavy exposure as well as melasma as they act on UV, visible and infrared spectrums and are opaque, providing a good camouflage effect (Box 2). But, these are messy, comedogenic, and there are concerns regarding free radical production. To prevent free radical production and whiteness, they are being formulated in micronized forms coated with dimethicone or silica.

Zinc oxide has greater protection in the UVA1 range. Micronized titanium dioxide shows synergistic effects with organic filters (Box 2).

Box 2: Inorganic sunscreens

- Zinc oxide
- Titanium oxide
- Magnesium oxide
- Iron oxide
- Red veterinary petrolatum

Organic Sunscreens

These are aromatic compounds with a carboxyl group that absorb UV light of a specific wavelength, and then emit a longer wavelength of lesser energy, usually in the form of insensible heat.[3,7,9,10] The molecule may structurally degrade because of the high energy state when it is labeled as photo-unstable[10] (Table 5).

Table 5: Organic UVB filters

USAN name	INCI name	Peak absorption wavelength
Aminobenzoates		
PABA	PABA	283 nm
Padimate O	Ethyl dimethyl PABA	311 nm
Cinnamates		
Octinoxate	Ethylhexyl methoxycinnamate	311 nm
Cinoxate	Cinoxate	289 nm
Salicylates		
Octisalate	Ethylhexyl salicylate	307 nm
Homosalate	Homosalate	306 nm
Trolamine salicylate	Time and extent application salicylate	260 nm, 355 nm
Benzophenones		
Others		
Octocrylene	Octocrylene	303 nm
Ensulizole	Phenylbenzimidazole sulfonic acid	310 nm
Mexoryl XL	DTS	303 nm, 344 nm

DTS, drometrizole trisiloxane; INCI, International Nomenclature Cosmetic Ingredient; PABA, para-aminobenzoic acid; USAN, United States Adopted Name.

Table 6: Organic ultraviolet A filters		
Class	**Name**	**Peak absorption wavelength**
Benzophenones		
Oxybenzone	Benzophenone 3	288 nm, 325 nm
Sulisobenzone	Benzophenone 4	366 nm
Dioxybenzone	Benzophenone 8	352 nm
Tinosorb M	MBBT	305 nm, 306 nm
Tinosorb S	BEMT	310 nm, 343 nm
Other		
Methylanthranilate	Meradimate	355 nm
Avobenzone/Parsol 1789	BMDM	360 nm
Mexoryl SX	TDSA	345 nm
Mexoryl XL	DTS	303 nm, 344 nm
Uvinul A plus	DHHB	354 nm
NeoHeliopan AP	DPDT	335 nm

BMDM, butyl methoxydibenzoylmethane; BMET, bis-ethylhexyloxyphenol methoxyphenyl triazine; DHHB, diethylamino hydroxybenzoyl hexyl benzoate; DPDT, disodium phenyl dibenzimidazole tetrasulfonat; DTS, drometrizole trisiloxane MBBT, methylene bis-benzotriazolyl tetramethylbutylphenol; TDSA, terephthalylidene dicamphor sulfonic acid.

There is a risk of contact dermatitis specially with benzophenones and PABA. Avobenzone and cinnamates are photo-unstable, and hence are combined with octocrylene and tinosorb S. Synergistic effect is shown by the combination of TDSA and DTS, and TDSA and BEMT[10] (Table 6).

Sunscreen Protection Criteria

There is much confusion and ignorance about judging the efficacy of sunscreens (Box 3).

Box 3: Criteria for evaluation of sunscreen protection

- SPF
- PA factor—Japanese standard
- Australian/New Zealand standard
- European union rating
- Boots star rating
- Critical wavelength

PA, protection grade of UVA; SPF, sunburn protection factor.

Sunburn Protection Factor

Sunburn protection factor (SPF) is defined as the ratio of the least amount of ultraviolet energy (UVB) required to produce minimal erythema dose (MED) on sunscreen protected skin to the amount of energy required to produce the same erythema on unprotected skin. About 2 mg/cm^2 layer of sunscreen is required to protect the skin.[2-4,6,7,9]

With chronic exposure, the damage caused by UV radiation is halved by a sunscreen having SPF30 compared to a sunscreen of SPF15.[2-4,7,9-11]

Products having SPF more than 50 can only write "SPF 50+" on the packaging.

PA Rating[12]

It is the ratio of the UVA dose required to produced PPD after 2–24 hours of exposure on protected skin to the UVA dose required to produce the same effect on unprotected skin. Since it measures the ability to prevent tanning, it is a more useful measure for darker skin types and patients of melasma (Table 7).

Table 7: PA rating according to degree of PPD ratio

PA	PPD ratio
+	2–4
++	4–8
+++	>8

PA, protection grade of UVA; PPD, persistent pigment darkening.

Australia/New Zealand Standard

This is an *in vitro* method in which an 8 μm layer of the product should not transmit more than 10% of the radiation and a 20 μm layer should not transmit more than 1% of the radiation of wavelength 320–360 nm.

European Standard

It states that SPF/UVA protection factor ratio should be less than or equal to 3.[13]

Boots Star Rating

This is an *in vitro* method, which is a measure of UVA protection, where UVA to UVB absorbance before and after irradiation is calculated as shown in table 8.

Table 8: Boots star rating

Before	After	Boots star rating
<0.6	<0.56	None
>0.6	>57	***
>0.8	>76	****
>0.9	>86	*****

Substantivity

Substantivity refers to the ability of a sunscreen to retain its effectiveness under the stress of exercise, sweating, and swimming.[3,9]

A sunscreen is labeled as water resistant if it is able to retain its efficacy after two sequential immersions in water for 20 minute each. A very water resistant sunscreen can do so after four sequential immersions. A water resistant sunscreen is also sweat resistant. The word water proof is not to be used.

Application of Sunscreens

A thick layer, ideally 2 mg/cm^2 should be applied for the sunscreen to be effective[3,9,14] (Table 9).

Table 9: The teaspoon rule	
3 mL or just more than half teaspoon	Each arm, face, and neck
5 mL or just more than one teaspoon	Each leg, chest, and back

Selecting the Right Sunscreen for a Patient with Melasma

The following points should be considered

- Inorganic sunscreens preferred as they have a broad spectrum covering UVA, UVB as visible spectrum and also provided camouflage effect as these are opaque.
- Since inorganic sunscreens alone are not cosmetically acceptable, blend with organic.
- Use liberally and repeatedly even when you are indoors
- Note the coexisting conditions, such as acne, occupation and the needs, and aspirations of the patient. Use a gel based preparation for acne patients, outdoor workers, and water in oil emulsion for aged and dry skin.

COSMETIC CAMOUFLAGE FOR MELASMA[15]

Cosmetic camouflage is a makeup used to conceal the skin discoloration and normalize the appearance of skin helping in improving self-esteem and quality of life. These products are different from foundations as they have 25% more pigment and also have fillers with optical properties. Indications vary from macular lesions to papules, nodules, scars, injuries, etc. (Boxes 4–7).

Box 4: Goals of cosmetic camouflage

- Match all skin tones and blend into the surrounding area
- Conceal adequately
- Water and sweat resistant
- Not slide off
- Stay for a sufficient time
- Be easy to apply

Box 5: Types of cosmetic camouflage

- Full concealment
- Pigment blending
- Subtle coverage

Box 6: Steps of cosmetic camouflage

- Ask the patient about previous experience
- Cleanse, exfoliate, and moisturize the area, preferably with a sunscreen
- Match the product to the patient's skin
- Identify underlying skin tones that are contributing to the skin color, e.g., hemoglobin—red, keratin—yellow, melanin—brown
- Understand color coordinates—hue*, value† and intensity‡

*Hue is the coordinate for the spectrum color, commonly the color name
†Value is the relative darkness or lightness
‡Intensity or chroma or saturation is the brightness

Box 7: Key points

- Difficult to match with a single color, so mix and match
- Watch out for manufacturer variation
- Judge on the skin, not in the container
- Different areas of the body may vary in color
- Keep tester kit
- Provide a mirror to the patient
- Photograph before and after
- Testing area should be well illuminated

CONCLUSION

Photoprotection forms the cornerstone of any therapeutic regimen for melasma, and increases the effectiveness of other therapeutic modalities. It helps in preventing synthesis of new melanin by melanocytes and helps in improving the overall and texture of the skin. Physicians should be aware of the various options available to them and choose a product wisely.

Editor's Note

Photoprotection, if used effectively, could play an important role in treatment of melasma. Visible light has a role to play in melasma, hence inorganic sunscreens are important. Cosmetic camouflage can improve the quality of life in patients with melasma.

REFERENCES

1. Matts PJ. Solar ultraviolet radiation: Definitions and terminology. Dermatol Clin. 2006; 24:1-8.
2. Lim HW. Photoprotection and sun-protective agents. In: Wolff K, Goldsmith LA, Katz SI, Gilchrest BA, Paller AS, Leffell DJ, editors. Fitzpatrick's Dermatology in General Medicine. 7th edition. New York: McGraw-Hill; 2008. pp. 2137-41.
3. Rai R, Srinivas CR. Photoprotection. Indian J Dermatol Venereol Leprol. 2007;73:73-9.
4. Moyal D. Need for a well-balanced sunscreen to protect human skin from both ultraviolet A and ultraviolet B damage. Indian J Dermatol Venereol Leprol. 2012;78:24-30.

5. Rai VM, Shenoi SD, Balachandran C, Pai S. Minimal erythema response (MED) to solar simulated irradiation in normal Indian skin. Indian J Dermatol Venereol Leprol. 2004;70:277-9.
6. Levy SB. Sunscreens. In: Wolverton SE, editor. Comprehensive dermatologic drug therapy, 2ndEdition. Philadelphia: WB Saunders; 2007. pp. 703-18.
7. Moyal D, Galdi A, Oresajo C. Sunscreens. In: Zoe Diana Draelos, editor. Cosmetic Dermatology Products and Procedures. New Jersey: Wiley-Blackwell; 2010. pp. 144-9.
8. Hexsel CL, Bangert SD, Hebert AA, Lim HW. Current sunscreen issues: 2007 Food and Drug Administration sunscreen labelling recommendations and combination sunscreen/ insect repellent products. J Am Acad Dermatol. 2008;59:316-23.
9. Kaimal S, Abraham A. Sunscreens. Indian J Dermatol Venereol Leprol. 2011;77:238-43.
10. Moyal D. The development of efficient sunscreens. Indian J Dermatol Venereol Leprol. 2012;78:31-4.
11. Moyal D. Prevention of ultraviolet-induced skin pigmentation. Photodermatol Photo-immunol Photomed. 2004;20:243-7.
12. Japan Cosmetic Industry Association (JCIA). Measurements standard for UVA protection efficacy. Tokyo, Japan: JCIA; 1996.
13. European Commission recommendation. On the efficacy of sunscreen products and the claims made relating thereto. Official J Eur Union. 2006;265:39-43.
14. Schneider J. The teaspoon rule of applying sunscreen. Arch Dermatol. 2002;138:838-9.
15. Bouloc Anne. Camouflage Techniques. In: Zoe Diana Draelos, editor. Cosmetic Dermatology Products and Procedures. New Jersey:Wiley-Blackwell; 2010. pp. 176-83.

CHAPTER 8

Hydroquinone Based Therapies for Melasma

Rashmi Sarkar, Shivani Bansal, Sumit Sethi

INTRODUCTION

Melasma is derived from the Greek word, *"melas"* meaning black. It is a common acquired pigmentary disorder of sun-exposed skin which presents as symmetric, light to dark brown colored patches having irregular, serrated, and geographic borders. Persons with dark skin are more susceptible, particularly those with Fitzpatrick skin types IV to VI, although patients with all skin types and ethnicities can develop melasma. It is more common in women, especially in their reproductive years, but about 10% cases occur in men. In an Indian study by Sarkar et al., 20.5% patients of melasma were men and no difference was noted clinically and histopathologically, as compared to melasma in females.[1]

Multiple risk factors and biological/environmental triggers have been implicated in the etiopathogenesis of melasma, including female sex, genetics, degree of exposure to solar radiation, pregnancy, oral contraceptives, hormonal therapies (e.g., estrogen-progesterone treatments), and photosensitizing medications. The three major patterns of distribution are: (1) centrofacial (cheeks, forehead, upper lip, nose, and chin) (66% of cases), (2) malar (cheeks and nose) (20% of cases), and (3) mandibular (rami of the mandible) (15% of cases). Histologically, the condition may be primarily epidermal, dermal, or mixed. Epidermal melasma is characterized by excess melanin deposition in basal, suprabasal, and stratum corneum layers, whereas dermal melasma exhibits melanophages in both the superficial and the deep dermis.

By causing cosmetic disfigurement of the face, melasma is frequently associated with significant emotional and psychological stress. The management of melasma is challenging and requires a long-term treatment plan. Topical therapy has remained the mainstay of treatment. Different therapeutic modalities, especially the gold standard hydroquinone (HQ) have been used in the topical treatment of melasma. The other modalities which are used are topical depigmenting agents, used alone, or in combinations and peeling agents like glycolic, trichloroacetic acid, salicylic, and lactic acid. Physical agents like lasers and dermabrasion have also been tried with limited success.[2] Because sun exposure is an important etiologic factor in hyperpigmentation, all patients should use, broad-spectrum, high SPF sunscreens and minimize sun exposure. Although clinical studies on their role are lacking.

This chapter focuses on HQ therapy in melasma, which could potentially be used as alone or in combination in treatment for melasma.

HYDROQUINONE

Hydroquinone, also known as dihydroxybenzene, is a hydroxyphenolic compound that is structurally similar to precursors of melanin. It inhibits the conversion of DOPA to melanin by inhibition of the enzyme, tyrosinase. Other proposed mechanisms are the inhibition of DNA and RNA synthesis, degradation of melanosomes and destruction of melanocytes.[3] Efficacy is directly linked to concentration, but the incidence of adverse effects also increases with concentration. HQ can be applied in cream form or as an alcohol-based solution.

Hydroquinone is very difficult to formulate in a stable preparation. It is a highly reactive oxidant that rapidly combines with oxygen. Typically, HQ skin-lightening creams are a creamy color that changes to a darker yellow or brown as oxidation occurs. As the discoloration progresses, the activity of the HQ decreases. Products with any off-color change should be immediately discarded.

Hydroquinone is the most frequently prescribed depigmenting agent worldwide and it has remained the gold standard for the treatment of melasma, particularly of the epidermal type. Variably good yet reversible results are obtained in most of the patients treated with HQ. The depigmenting effects of the HQ treatment become evident after 5–7 weeks. Treatment should be continued for at least 3 months, up to 1 year. HQ is also formulated in combination with other agents like, topical steroids, retinoids, kojic acid (KA), and glycolic acids (GAs) for added benefits.

MONOTHERAPY

It is used as monotherapy in concentrations of 2–5%, though 4% is the preferred one especially in the Indian setup. In a double-blind placebo-controlled trial involving 48 patients with melasma on the face, HQ 4% or placebo was applied twice daily for 12 weeks. Results indicated total improvement of melasma in 40% of patients treated with HQ and there was no treatment failures. In contrast, in the placebo group, 10% of patients had total improvement, but 20% were classified as treatment failures.[4]

COMBINATIONS

Hydroquinone can be combined with tretinoin and steroid as triple combination therapy or can also be used in conjunction with chemical peels.

RETINOID WITH HYDROQUINONE

Retinoids, such as tretinoin, is thought to have an inhibitory effect on tyrosinase by inhibiting the enzyme's transcription, as well as on dopachrome conversion factor, with a resulting interruption of melanin synthesis and also reduces hyperpigmentation through the induction of desquamation.[5] Compared with phenolic compounds like HQ, it typically takes at least 24 weeks with retinoid to see clinical improvement. Retinoid acid (RA) concentrations ranging from 0.05% to 0.1% have been used. RA 0.1% plus 3% HQ has been evaluated in 40 female Korean women in a 20-week open label study. Overall, 59% of patients were rated as having excellent to good improvement by physician and patient evaluations after therapy. The majority of patients (96%) noted mild to moderate reactions to tretinoin cream. The sensations of burning, itching, erythema, and scaliness lessened with continued therapy.[6]

Glycolic Acid with Hydroquinone

Glycolic acid 5–12% is an α-hydroxy acid and has been studied in combination with other agents. It decreases pigment by many mechanisms including thinning the stratum corneum, enhancing epidermolysis, dispersing melanin in the basal layer of the epidermis, and increasing collagen synthesis in the dermis.

In a randomized controlled trial, 10% GA plus 4% HQ in a cream containing vitamins C and E and sunscreen was compared with a cream containing sunscreen alone in group of Hispanic patients. Results indicated a significant decrease in the degree of pigmentation using the study cream compared with sunscreen alone; ($p = 0.001$). Irritation was a common side effect which resolved with the temporary cessation of application and application of moisturizers.[7]

Kojic Acid and Hydroquinone

Kojic acid 2% is produced by the fungus *Aspergilline oryzae*. It also inhibits tyrosinase and is also a potent antioxidant. Kojic acid may be used if a patient has difficulty tolerating other first-line therapies. It is used concentrations ranging from 1% to 4% and has been found equivalent to other therapies but may cause more irritation. In a study, KA in synergy with HQ 2% is a superior depigmenting agent as compared to KA alone or with its combinations with 0.1% betamethasone valerate or a combination of 0.1% betamethasone valerate and HQ 2%. [8]

Triple Combination Therapy

The preferred topical application is in the form of triple combination (TC) where HQ is used along with a topical steroid and a retinoid. The addition of tretinoin eliminates pigment and increases keratinocyte proliferation by preventing the oxidation of HQ and improving epidermal penetration. Further, adding topical corticosteroids reduces the irritant effects of hypopigmenting agents, and inhibits melanin synthesis by decreasing cellular metabolism. This combination of HQ 5%, tretinoin 0.1%, and dexamethasone 0.1%, was first introduced in 1975 and termed as the Kligman formula (KF) after its inventor. It has been the most extensively used combination therapy for melasma worldwide in various different combinations and modifications.[9]

Taylor et al. compared the efficacy and safety of a hydrophilic cream formulation containing tretinoin 0.05%, hydroquinone 4.0%, and fluocinolone acetonide 0.01% (RA+HQ+FA) with the dual-combination agents tretinoin plus hydroquinone (RA+HQ), tretinoin plus fluocinolone acetonide (RA+FA), and hydroquinone plus fluocinolone acetonide (HQ+FA) in a multicenter, randomized, investigator-blind study in 641 adult patients of moderate to severe melasma in Fitzpatrick skin types I–IV.[10] It was found that significantly more of the patients treated with RA+HQ+FA (26.1%) experienced complete clearing compared with the other treatment groups (4.6%) at the end of week 8 ($p < 0.0001$) and also 75% reduction in pigmentation was observed in more than 70% of patients treated with RA+HQ+FA compared with 30% in patients treated with the dual-combination agents.

Amongst the medical therapies analyzed by a recent Cochrane review, TC creams have been found to be the best topical therapy.[11] In a recent multicentered trial by Chan et al., 260 South East Asian patients were randomized to TC (FA 0.01%, HQ 4%, RA 0.05%) cream or 4% HQ cream for 8 weeks. Significantly more participants in the TC group (87/125) compared to the 4% HQ group (57/129) achieved a score of 0 (clear) or 1 (minor hyperpigmentation).[12] A similar study on 120 patients demonstrated significantly lower melasma severity scores in the triple therapy groups than in the HQ group.[13]

Triple combination cream exhibits a safe profile with low potential for adverse events. In a long-term, multicenter, open-label, study in 173 patients of once-daily application of TC therapy (FA 0.01%, HQ 4%, RA 0.05%), no cases of skin atrophy or skin thinning were seen after 6–12 months of treatment (one or two course). Only six cases showed telangiectasia, most of which had improved by the end of the study. Most adverse effects were expected: application-site reactions, that were mild and transient in nature and did not require remedial therapy.[14] In an another study of same TC combination for 24 weeks in 62 patients with moderate to severe melasma, the atrophogenic potential of TC cream was evaluated through serial histopathologic examination of skin biopsies. No significant histopathologic signs of atrophy of the epidermis or dermis were noted at any time point throughout the study.[15] To maintain safety profile, TC creams can be used continuously for 12 weeks then can be maintained twice per week for another 12 weeks if no relapse occurs.[16]

Triple combination creams can be combined with chemical peels or used as priming agents before chemical peels. Forty Indian patients with Fitzpatrick skin types III–IV with moderate to severe melasma were randomized to treatment with the modified Kligman's formula (hydrocortisone 1%, HQ 2%, tretinoin 0.05%) daily plus six serial GA 30–40% (chemical peel) treatments at 3-week intervals or to modified KF alone.[17] A significant decrease in the melasma area and severity index (MASI) score at 21 weeks compared with baseline was observed in both groups. But the group receiving GA showed a trend toward more rapid and greater improvements than the other group.

Others

A recent study in 15 Latin American women incorporated hyaluronic acid with HQ and GA as a novel cream preparation and found it to be well tolerated and with a significant decrease in MASI scores of 64% at the end of study in the treatment of melasma.[18]

ADVERSE REACTIONS

Adverse reactions of HQ are related to its dose and the duration of treatment. Irritation is the most common complication; other adverse effects include erythema, stinging, colloid milium, irritant and allergic contact dermatitis, nail discoloration, transient hypochromia, and paradoxical postinflammatory hypermelanosis. Prolonged use of HQ can result in blue black pigmentation of treated areas known as ochronosis. There was a proposed ban on HQ in 2006 due to concerns of ochronosis and carcinogenicity, but subsequently it was observed that the evidence of carcinogenicity due to topical application in human beings was not substantial.

Under no circumstances should monobenzyl ether, or any other ethers of HQ, be used to treat melasma as they can lead to a permanent loss of melanocytes with the development of a disfiguring confetti-like leukoderma.

Hydroquinone and Controversy

There are several important health issues that need to be considered before determining the safety of HQ. For many years, it has been known that HQ can cause ochronosis. Whether this is a result of the effect of HQ alone or other substances present in the formulation or higher concentrations of HQ is unknown. Additional concern arose when oral HQ was reported to cause cancer in rodents fed with large amounts of the substance, yet human carcinogenicity has not been established. Although oral consumption probably is not related to topical application, HQ remains controversial because it maybe toxic to melanocytes. Issues regarding the topical toxicity of HQ arise because it is a strong oxidant which gets rapidly converted to the melanocyte toxic products, p-benzoquinone and hydroxybenzoquinone. These by-products may cause depigmentation.[19]

Regulatory agencies in Japan, Europe, and most recently the United States of America, have raised questions about the safety of HQ and it has been banned in cosmetic preparations and OTC products in some countries. This has encouraged research into alternative agents for the topical management of melasma. However, despite 40–50 years use of hydroquinone for medical conditions, there has not been a single documented case of either a cutaneous or internal malignancy associated with this drug.[20] Modified Kligman regime is still used as first line treatment for melasma by dermatologists all over the world. The various therapies along with their level and quality of evidence are given in tables 1 and 2.

CONCLUSION

Melasma is a relatively common form of hyperpigmentation. There is no cure and the condition tends to recur; therefore, precautions need to be taken. The standard therapy for melasma is HQ, either as monotherapy or, more often, in combination with other agents such as topical corticosteroids and tretinoin. Fixed triple combination or modified Kligman's regime is time tested and remains first line treatment even though there are so many newer skin lightening agents and cosmeceuticals. Supervised use under the direction of a dermatologist is good for the patient.

Table 1: Quality and level of evidence	
Quality of evidence	
I	Evidence obtained from at least one properly designed, randomized control trial
II-i	Evidence obtained from well designed controlled trials without randomization
II-ii	Evidence obtained from well designed cohort or case control analytic studies, preferably from more than one center or research group
II-iii	Evidence obtained from multiple time series with or without the intervention. Dramatic results in uncontrolled experiments (such as the results of the introduction of penicillin in the 1940s) could also be regarded as this type of evidence
III	Opinions of respected authorities based on clinical experience, descriptive studies, or reports of expert committees
IV	Evidence inadequate owing to problems of methodology (e.g., sample size, length, or comprehensiveness of follow-up or conflicts in evidence)
Level of evidence	
A	There is good evidence to support the use of this procedure
B	There is fair evidence to support the use of this procedure
C	There is poor evidence to support the use of the procedure
D	There is fair evidence to support the rejection of the use of the procedure
E	There is good evidence to support the rejection of the use of this procedure

Table 2: Level and quality of evidence for melasma therapies

		Therapy	Level of evidence	Quality of evidence
Epidermal melasma	Topical	2% HQ[21]	II-ii	C
		4% HQ[4,22-24]	I	B
		4% HQ + 0.05% RA + 0.01% fluocinolone acetonide[10,14,20,25]	I	A
		20% Azelaic acid[21,22]	I	B
		0.05% RA[14]	I	C
		Adapalene[26]	II-ii	B
		Kojic acid[27,28]	II-i	B
		Vitamin C[29]	I	B
	Chemical peels	10%-50% GA[30]	II-ii/II-iii	C
		70% GA[31]	II-i	B
		Jessner's solution[31]	II-i	C
		20%-30% salicylic acid[32,33]	II-iii/III	C
		Lactic acid[34]	II-iii	C
		1%-5% RA[35]	III	C
	Derma-abrasion[36]		II-iii	E
	Broad spectrum sun protection[37,38]		II-i/II-iii	B

Continued

Continued

Table 2: Level and quality of evidence for melasma therapies				
Dermal melasma	Lasers	Pulsed CO_2 laser followed by Q-switched alexandrite laser[39]	IV	C
		Q switched ruby laser[40]	II-iii	C
		Erbium:YAG laser	II-iii	D
		Fractional laser resurfacing[41,42]	II-iii	C
		Intense pulsed light[43,44]	II-iii	C
		Copper Bromide[45]	II-iii	C

GA, glycolic acid; HQ, hydroquinone; KA, kojic acid; KF, Kligman's formula; RA, retinoic acid; TCA, trichloroacetic acid.

Editor's Note

Inspite of so many newer and promising agents for melasma, topical hydroquinone and modified Kligman's therapy remain the most efficacious therapy for melasma, if used judiciously. Of course, one needs to monitor side effects and look for erythema, darkening- or pepper-like appearance to stop therapy.

REFERENCES

1. Sarkar R, Puri P, Jain RK, Singh A, Desai A. Melasma in men: A clinical, aetiological and histological study. J Eur Acad Dermatol Venereol. 2010;24:768-72.
2. Rendon M, Berneburg M, Arellano I, Picardo M. Treatment of melasma. J Am Acad Dermatol. 2006;54:S272-81.
3. Jimbow K, Obata H, Pathak MA, Fitzpatrick TB. Mechanism of depigmentation by hydroquinone. J Invest Dermatol. 1974;62:436-49.
4. Ennes SBP, Paschoalick RC, Mota De Avelar Alchorne M. A double-blind, comparative, placebo-controlled study of the efficacy and tolerability of 4% hydroquinone as a depigmenting agent in melasma. J Dermatolog Treat. 2000;11:173-9.
5. Roméro C, Aberdam E, Larnier C, Ortonne JP. Retinoic acid as modulator of UVB-induced melanocyte differentiation. Involvement of the melanogenic enzymes expression. J Cell Sci. 1994;107:1095-103.
6. Kauh YC, Zachian TF. Melasma. Adv Exp Med Biol. 1999;455:491-9.
7. Guevara IL, Pandya AG. Safety and efficacy of 4% hydroquinone combined with 10% glycolic acid, antioxidants, and sunscreen in the treatment of melasma. Int J Dermatol. 2003;42:966-72.
8. Deo KS, Dash KN, Sharma YK, Virmani NC, Oberai C. Kojic Acid vis-a-vis its Combinations with Hydroquinone and Betamethasone Valerate in Melasma: A Randomized, Single Blind, Comparative Study of Efficacy and Safety. Indian J Dermatol. 2013 Jul;58:281-5.
9. Kligman AM, Willis I. A new formula for depigmenting human skin. Arch Dermatol. 1975;111:40-8.
10. Taylor SC, Torok H, Jones T, Lowe N, Rich P, Tschen E, et al. Efficacy and safety of a new triple-combination agent for the treatment of facial melasma. Cutis. 2003;72(1):67-72.
11. Jutley GS, Rajaratnam R, Halpern J, Salim A, Emmett C. Systematic review of randomized controlled trials on interventions for melasma: an abridged Cochrane review. J Am Acad Dermatol. 2014;70:369-73.

12. Chan R, Park KC, Lee MH, Lee ES, Chang SE, Leow YH, et al. A randomized controlled trial of the efcacy and safety of a xed triple combination (uocinolone acetonide 0.01%, hydroquinone 4%, tretinoin 0.05%) compared with hydroquinone 4% cream in Asian patients with moderate to severe melasma. Br J Dermatol. 2008;159:697-703.
13. Ferreira Cestari T, Hassun K, Sittart A, de Lourdes Viegas M. A comparison of triple combination cream and hydroquinone 4% cream for the treatment of moderate to severe facial melasma. J Cosmet Dermatol. 2007;6:36-9.
14. Torok HM, Jones T, Rich P, Smith S, Tschen E. Hydroquinone 4%, tretinoin 0.05%, fluocinolone acetonide 0.01%: a safe and efficacious 12-month treatment for melasma. Cutis. 2005;75:57-62.
15. Bhawan J, Grimes P, Pandya AG, Keady M, Byers HR, Guevara IL, et al. A histological examination for skin atrophy after 6 months of treatment with fluocinolone acetonide 0.01%, hydroquinone 4%, and tretinoin 0.05% cream. Am J Dermatopathol. 2009;31: 794-8.
16. Grimes PE, Bhawan J, Guevara IL, Colón LE, Johnson LA, Gottschalk RW, et al. Continuous therapy followed by a maintenance therapy regimen with a triple combination cream for melasma. J Am Acad Dermatol. 2010;62:962-7.
17. Sarkar R, Kaur C, Bhalla M, Kanwar AJ. The combination of glycolic acid peels with a topical regimen in the treatment of melasma in dark-skinned patients: a comparative study. Dermatol Surg. 2002;28:828-32.
18. Guevara IL, Werlinger KD, Pandya AG. Tolerability and efficacy of a novel formulation in the treatment of melasma. J Drugs Dermatol. 2010;9:215-8.
19. Draelos ZD. Skin lightening preparations and the hydroquinone controversy. Dermatol Ther. 2007;20:308-13.
20. Nordlund JJ, Grimes PE, Ortonne JP. The safety of hydroquinone. J Eur Acad Dermatol Venereol. 2006;20:781-7.
21. Verallo-Rowell VM, Verallo V, Graupe K, Lopez-Villafuerte L, Garcia-Lopez M. Double-blind comparison of azelaic acid and hydroquinone in the treatment of melasma. Acta Derm Venereol Suppl (Stockh). 1989;143:58-61.
22. Balina LM, Graupe K. The treatment of melasma. 20% azelaic acid versus 4% hydroquinone cream. Int J Dermatol. 1991;30:893-5.
23. Amer M, Metwalli M. Topical hydroquinone in the treatment of some hyperpigmentary disorders. Int J Dermatol. 1998;37:449-50.
24. Haddad AL, Matos LF, Brunstein F, Ferreira LM, Silva A, Costa D. A clinical, prospective, randomized, double-blind trial comparing skin whitening complex with hydroquinone vs. placebo in the treatment of melasma. Int J Dermatol. 2003;42:153-6.
25. Cestari T, Adjadj L, Hux M, Shimizu MR, Rives VP. Cos-effectiveness of a fixed combination of hydroquinone/ tretinoin/fluocinolone cream compared with hydroquinone alone in the treatment of melasma. J Drugs Dermatol. 2007;6:153-60.
26. Dogra S, Kanwar AJ, Parsad D. Adapalene in the treatment of melasma: a preliminary report. J Dermatol. 2002;29:539-40.
27. Lim JT. Treatment of melasma using kojic acid in a gel containing hydroquinone and glycolic acid. Dermatol Surg. 1999;25:282-4.
28. Garcia A, Fulton JE Jr. The combination of glycolic acid and hydroquinone or kojic acid for the treatment of melasma and related conditions. Dermatol Surg. 1996;22:443-7.
29. Espinal-Perez LE, Moncada B, Castanedo-Cazarez JP. A double-blind randomized trial of 5% ascorbic acid vs. 4% hydroquinone in melasma. Int J Dermatol. 2004;43:604-7.
30. Javaheri SM, Handa S, Kaur I, Kumar B. Safety and efficacy of glycolic acid facial peel in Indian women with melasma. Int J Dermatol. 2001;40:354-7.
31. Lawrence N, Cox SE, Brody HJ. Treatment of melasma with Jessner's solution versus glycolic acid: a comparison of clinical efficacy and evaluation of the predictive ability of Wood's light examination. J Am Acad Dermatol. 1997;36:589-93.
32. Grimes PE. The safety and efficacy of salicylic acid chemical peels in darker racial-ethnic groups. Dermatol Surg. 1999;25: 18-22.

33. Hyo HA, Kim I-H. Whitening effect of salicylic acid peels in Asian patients. Dermatol Surg. 2006;32:372-5.
34. Sharquie KE, Al-Tikreety MM, Al-Mashhadani SA. Lactic acid as a new therapeutic peeling agent in melasma. Dermatol Surg. 2005;31:149-54.
35. Cuce´ LC, Bertino MC, Scattone LK, Birkenhauer MC. Tretinoin peeling. Dermatol Surg. 2001;27:12-4.
36. Kunachak S, Leelaudomlipi P, Wongwaisayawan S. Dermabrasion: a curative treatment for melasma. Aesthetic Plast Surg. 2001;25:114-7.
37. Lakhdar H, Zouhair K, Khadir K, Essari A, Richard A, Seite S, et al. Evaluation of the effectiveness of broad-spectrum sunscreen in the prevention of chloasma in pregnant women. J Eur Acad Dermatol Venereol. 2007;21:738-42.
38. Vázquez M, Sánchez JL. The efficacy of a broad-spectrum sunscreen in the treatment of melasma. Cutis. 1983;32:92, 95-6.
39. Nouri K, Bowes L, Chartier T, Romagosa R, Spencer J. Combination treatment of melasma with pulsed CO2 laser followed by Q-switched alexandrite laser: a pilot study. Dematol Surg. 1999;25:494-7.
40. Taylor CR, Anderson RR. Ineffective treatment of refractory melasma and postinflammatory hyperpigmentation by Q-switched ruby laser. J Dermatol Surg Oncol. 1994;20:592-7.
41. Rokhsar CK, Fitzpatrick RE. The treatment of melasma with fractional photothermolysis: a pilot study. Dermatol Surg. 2005;31:1645-50.
42. Goldberg DJ, Berlin AL, Phelps R. Histologic and ultrastructural analysis of melasma after fractional resurfacing. Lasers Surg Med. 2008;40:134-8.
43. Li Y-H, Chen JZS, Wei H-C, Wu Y, Liu M, Xu YY, et al. Efficacy and safety of intense pulsed light in treatment of melasma in Chinese patients. Dermatol Surg. 2008;34:693-701.
44. Wang CC, Hui CY, Sue YM, Wong WR, Hong HS. Intense pulsed light for the treatment of refractory melasma in Asian persons. Dermatol Surg. 2004;30:1196-200.
45. Lee HI, Lim YY, Kim BJ, Kim MN, Min HJ, Hwang JH, et al. Clinicopathologic efficacy of copper bromide plus/yellow laser(578 nm with 511 nm) for treatment of melasma in Asian patients. Dermatol Surg. 2010;36:885-93.

CHAPTER 9

Non-Hydroquinone Based Therapies for Melasma

Latika Arya

INTRODUCTION

Melasma is a chronic and recurring disorder of pigmentation, causing significant psychosocial impairment. The treatment is challenging, prolonged, and requires a judicious approach especially in dark skinned patients. Hydroquinone (HQ) although quite efficacious, may have significant side effects including skin irritation, contact dermatitis and exogenous ochronosis. Hence there is a growing need for alternative natural, safe, and efficacious skin lightening agents. Recent studies show that several non-hydroquinone agents may also play an important role in therapy for hyperpigmentation.[1] These agents selectively target hyperplastic melanocytes and inhibit key regulatory steps in melanogenesis. The various non-hydroquinone skin lightening agents can be classified into four major groups based on their mechanism of action (Table 1).

1. Tyrosinase inhibition.
2. Inhibition of melanosome transfer.
3. Increased turnover of epidermis.
4. Anti-inflammatory and antioxidant effects.

Non-hydroquinone agents are reviewed here, with a focus on those that have clinical trial findings, supporting their efficacy.

Table 1: Mechanism of action of non-hydroquinone skin lightening agents

Mechanism of action	Skin lightening agents
Competitive tyrosinase inhibition	Azelaic acid, arbutin, deoxyarbutin, aloesin, kojic acid, flavonoids, gentisic acid, mequinol
Non-competitive tyrosinase inhibition	Glabridin, hydroxystilbenes (resveratrol, genitol), N-acetyl glucosamine
Inhibition of melanosomal transfer	Niacinamide, soy (soybean trypsin inhibitors)
Antioxidant	Vitamin C, vitamin E
Acceleration of epidermal turnover and desquamation	α-hydroxy acids, salicylic acid, linoleic acid, and retinoic acids

NON-HYDROQUINONE SKIN LIGHTENING PRODUCTS AGENTS

Kojic Acid

Kojic acid (KA) is a naturally occurring fungal metabolite derived from certain species of *Aspergillus, Acetobacter,* and *Penicillium*. It reduces hyperpigmentation by tyrosinase inhibition by binding to copper. It is the most popular non-hydroquinone agent employed for the treatment of melasma.[2]

Kojic acid is used at concentrations ranging from 1% to 4%. Although KA alone is less effective than HQ 2%, combination with glycolic acid (GA) 10% and HQ 2% augments efficacy.[3] Addition of KA may be beneficial in patients who do not respond to HQ, as seen in a 12-week, split-face, randomized study of 40 Chinese women with melasma, wherein 2% KA in a gel containing 10% GA and 2% HQ had a greater improvement as compared to the same combination without KA.[3] In another split-face study of 39 patients, 2% KA/5% GA and a 2% HQ/5% GA had an equal efficacy in lightening of pigmentation, including melasma.[4]

However, KA is a known sensitizer and has been shown to be mutagenic in cell culture studies.

Azelaic Acid

Azelaic acid is a naturally occurring dicarboxylic acid, obtained from *Pityrosporum* cultures, and associated with the hypomelanosis in *tinea versicolor*. It is a reversible inhibitor of tyrosinase activity and has an antiproliferative and cytotoxic effect on abnormal melanocytes.[5]

Azelaic acid 15–20% has been found to be of equivalent efficiency to HQ 4% in the treatment of melasma, and postinflammatory hyperpigmentation.[4] Combinations with topical tretinoin 0.05% and GA 15–20% are synergistic.[4]

Azelaic acid has an excellent safety profile but may cause transient erythema, stinging, pruritus, scaling, and allergic sensitization on rare occasions.

This is, according to the editor, a wonderful product to use if one is intolerant to fixed triple combination cream.

Arbutin

Arbutin is one of the most widely prescribed skin lightening and depigmenting agents worldwide. Arbutin is a naturally occurring D-glucopyranoside derivative of HQ found in bearberry leaves that converts to HQ *in vivo*. It competitively inhibits tyrosinase and 5,6-dihydroxyindole-2-carboxylic acid polymerase activities in a dose dependent manner in cultured melanocytes.[1] It also inhibits melanosome maturation and is less cytotoxic to melanocytes than HQ. Higher concentrations may be more efficacious, albeit with a risk of paradoxical hyperpigmentation. Studies show that arbutin is less effective than KA for hyperpigmentation. However, α-arbutin and deoxyarbutin, the synthetic derivate of arbutin, have a higher efficacy and stability in comparison to arbutin.[2,4] An *in vitro* comparative trial showed that HQ, arbutin, and deoxyarbutin had similar inhibitory effects on tyrosinase activity.[6] In a clinical study, topical treatment with deoxyarbutin for 12 weeks resulted in a significant reduction in overall skin lightness and improvement in solar lentigines in a population of light-skinned or dark-skinned individuals, respectively.[6]

Soy

Soy contains active ingredients like isoflavones, vitamin E, and serine protease inhibitors-soybean trypsin inhibitor and Bowman-Birk protease inhibitor. The protease inhibitors inhibit proteinase-activated receptor 2 (PAR-2) activation, thereby inhibiting melanosome transfer.[2]

Furthermore, they have been shown to reduce ultraviolet B (UVB)-induced pigmentation.[4] The inhibition of melanosome transfer is reversible, thus its safety profile is excellent.

Total soy extract was found to have a mean 12% reduction in dyspigmentation in 14 out of 16 Latin women after 3 months.[4] A double-blind, placebo-controlled, 12-week clinical study of soy-containing moisturizer with broad-spectrum sunscreen (SPF 30) in 68 patients demonstrated significant improvements in the fine lines, mottled hyperpigmentation, blotchiness, and skin clarity at week 12.[4]

Niacinamide

Niacinamide is the biologically active amide of vitamin B3 and is found in many root vegetables and yeasts. It inhibits the transfer of melanosomes to keratinocytes thereby reducing pigmentation.[1] In a randomized, split-face study of 18 Asian women with hyperpigmentation, 5% niacinamide applied for 4 weeks significantly decreased the hyperpigmentation as compared to vehicle.[4] In another randomized, split-face study comparing niacinamide 4% cream with 4% HQ cream in the treatment of melasma (n = 27), similar colorimetric improvement was seen in both the study groups at 8 weeks.[4]

Licorice Extract

It comes from the root of *Glycyrrhiza glabra*. Its main component is glabridin, a tyrosinase inhibitor that was shown to reduce UVB irradiation induced pigmentation and erythema in guinea pigs when applied for 3 weeks.[4] It also exerts anti-inflammatory effects by inhibiting superoxide anion and cyclo-oxygenase activity.[1] Liquirtin, another component of licorice, induces skin lightening by dispersing melanin.[2]

A 20% liquiritin cream applied twice daily for 4 weeks yielded a reduction in pigmentation in a double-blind, controlled, split-face study of 20 women with melasma.[4]

Vitamin C

Vitamin C works by inhibiting tyrosinase activity through interacting with copper. It acts as a reducing agent at various oxidative steps of melanin formation, hence inhibiting melanogenesis. However, it is rapidly oxidized and is of limited stability. Hence, stable esterified derivatives have been developed like magnesium ascorbyl phosphate (MAP), ascorbyl 6-palmitate, and tetrahexyldecyl ascorbate.[1] In a study of 34 Asian patients of melasma or solar lentigines, using magnesium-

L-ascorbyl-2phosphate, 19 demonstrated significant lightening, as measured by colorimetry.[4] A study comparing 5% ascorbic acid and 4% HQ in 16 female patients with melasma found 62.5% and 93% improvement, respectively. Side effects were present in 68.7% with HQ versus 6.2% with ascorbic acid. Thus, although HQ showed better response, vitamin C may play a role as it is devoid of any side effects, either alone or in combination therapy.[1]

Vitamin E (α-Tocopherol Acetate)

Vitamin E (α-tocopherol acetate) has been shown to cause depigmentation by interference with lipid peroxidation of melanocyte membranes, increase in intracellular glutathione content, and inhibition of tyrosinase.[1] It also has photo-protective effects. It is often formulated together with vitamin C for its lightening effect.

A clinical double-blinded study showed a significant improvement of melasma and pigmented contact dermatitis lesions using topical vitamins E and C, with the combination showing better results compared to the single-vitamin treatment groups.[1] Topical α-tocopherol is mostly used at concentration of 5% or less. Side effects such as allergic or irritant reactions may be rarely seen.

Retinoids

Retinoids cause inhibition of tyrosinase and epidermal melanin dispersion. They also interfere with pigment transfer to keratinocytes and accelerate pigment loss by enhancing the epidermal cell turnover. They allow increased access to other pigment-lightening agents. The prescription retinoids used for direct improvement in skin pigmentation are tretinoin and tazarotene. Tretinoin applied in 38 patients with melasma over a 40 week period showed 68% improvement. However, side effects in the form of erythema and desquamation were seen in 88% patients.[7] Retinol is not as effective as tretinoin or tazarotene in pigment lightening but is less irritating.[2]

NEWER PRODUCTS

A number of synthetic and botanical compounds derived from natural sources are being investigated for their potential role in reducing melanin production and pigmentation. Although many of them are still in the experimental/research trial phase, a few salient ones which show possible benefits are mentioned below. They could potentially be used as treatment for melasma after their role is established by larger, well-designed clinical trials in future.

Aloesin

It is a low-molecular-weight glycoprotein obtained from aloe tree. It competitively inhibits tyrosinase and also tyrosine hydroxylase and 3,4-dihydroxyphenylalanine (DOPA) oxidase.[6] Because of its hydrophilic nature, its penetration is limited and hence is commonly used in combination with arbutin or deoxyarbutin for a synergistic effect.

N-Acetylglucosamine (Chitin)

N-acetylglucosamine (NAG) is an amino monosaccharide that works by inhibiting the conversion of pro-tyrosinase to tyrosinase.[4] In a 10-week, double-blind, vehicle-controlled study of 202 women, a moisturizer with 2% NAG and niacinamide demonstrated significant improvement in reducing areas of facial spots and the appearance of hyperpigmentation.[4]

Rucinol (4-n Butyl Resorcinol)

It is a phenolic derivative, which inhibits both tyrosinase and tyrosinase-related protein. In a prospective, double-blind, randomized, vehicle-controlled, split-face comparative trial of 32 female patients with melasma, a statistically significant lightening was seen with rucinol serum 0.3% applied twice daily for 12 weeks, after a 12-week follow-up.[8] A recent formulation of rucinol, as 0.1% liposomal cream, has an improved stability and enhanced penetration.[8]

Octadecenedioic Acid

It is a dicarboxylic acid with structural similarity to azelaic acid. Its skin whitening effects are mediated by the stimulation of peroxisome proliferator-activated receptors (PPARs), which are nuclear receptors modulating synthesis of tyrosinase mRNA. In a comparative study on 21 Chinese volunteers, 1% octadecenedioic acid cream applied on forearm for 8 weeks with a further follow-up of 4 weeks showed lightening up to 11% in 90% of individuals as compared to 2% arbutin applied on the other forearm.[8]

Flavonoids

These are benzopyrene derivatives, which can be classified into flavones, flavanols, isoflavones, flavanones, and anthocyanidins. They exert a potent antioxidant and anti-inflammatory action and act as a substrate competitor for the tyrosinases. They inhibit pigment induced by DOPA oxidation as shown in an *in vitro* comparative study.[8]

Coffeeberry Extract

It has anti-oxidant properties. Application of coffeeberry extract for 6 weeks improved hyperpigmentation in 40 patients with photo-damage.[1]

Mulberry Extract

It is derived from the root bark of the plant *Morus alba* L and contains flavonoids including mulberroside F. It is found to have skin lightening effect due to inhibition of tyrosinase and superoxide scavenging activity. IC50 (concentration causing 50% inhibition of activity of tyrosinase) is very low (0.396%) as compared to 5.5% for HQ and 10.0% for KA.[1] In a randomized controlled trial on 50 patients of melasma, mulberry extract was compared with vehicle and was found to have significant improvement in melasma area and severity index (MASI) score, average mexameter measurements, and QOL scores in treatment group.[9]

Tranexamic Acid: Trans-4 (Aminomethyl) Cyclohexane Carboxylic Acid

It is a lysine analog. It decreases α-melanocyte stimulating hormone by its antiplasmin activity, thus reducing melanin synthesis. In a study on 100 Korean women with melasma, tranexamic acid given intradermally (4 mg/mL) every week for 12 weeks caused significant decrease in MASI score ($p < 0.05$), and 76.5% subjects reported lightening of melasma with minimal side effects.[8] Tranexamic acid emulsion applied on 25 melasma patients for 5–18 weeks produced marked subjective improvement in 80% subjects within 8 weeks without any significant side effects.[8]

Orchid Extract

It has antioxidant activity and efficacy is similar to vitamin C in melasma and lentigines, as shown in a study comparing orchid extract to 3% vitamin C derivative in 48 female patients.[1]

Pycnogenol

It is obtained from the bark of French maritime pine *Pinus pinaster*. Its main constituents are procyanidins, polyphenolic monomers, phenolic, or cinnamic acids. It has antioxidant and anti-inflammatory properties. Oral pycnogenol has been found to reduce melasma severity although, studies on topical use are lacking.[1]

Boswellia (Boswellic Acids)

They are pentacyclic triterpenes, extracted from the gum resins of the tropical tree *Boswellia serrata*. Boswellic acids are found to exert significant anti-inflammatory and pro-apoptotic activity as determined by several *in vitro* studies and clinical trials.[1]

Epigallocatechin-3-Gallate

It is obtained from green tea leaves and has been demonstrated to modulate melanin production in dose-dependent manner and also possesses anti-inflammatory properties.[8] However, more *in vivo* studies are needed to substantiate this action.

Ellagic Acid

It is isolated from green tea, eucalyptus, and strawberry and found to inhibit tyrosinase activity in B16 melanoma cells comparable to arbutin. In an open label randomized controlled trial on 30 patients of melasma, combination of plant derived and synthetic ellagic acid was compared with arbutin and significant improvement in pigment density was found on Mexameter in all groups with no statistical difference between them.[9]

Hesperidin

It is a bioflavonoid present in citrus fruits. Its structure is similar to that of HQ. It inhibits tyrosinase activity in melanoma B16 cells and human primary melanocytes and suppresses ultraviolet A induced damage of fibroblasts and oxidative damage of collagen.[10]

Hydroxystilbene Compounds

Resveratrol is one common example, shown to reduce not only tyrosinase activity but also MITF expression in B16 mouse melanoma cells.[6]

Gentisic Acid

It is derived from gentian roots. Its alkyl ester, especially methyl gentisate, is a highly effective skin lightening agent and less cytotoxic than HQ.[8]

Silymarin

It is a naturally occurring polyphenol flavonoid compound derived from thistle plant *Silybum marianum*, which has tyrosinase inhibitory and antioxidant effects.[8] In a randomized controlled trial on 96 subjects, it showed significant improvements in macule size, MASI scores, and physician assessments as compared to vehicle.[9]

Alpha Lipoic Acid/Thioctic Acid/Dihydrolipoic Acid

It is a disulfide derivative of octanoic acid. Its combination product with zinc—sodium zinc dihydrolipoyl histidinate has been studied by Tsuji Naito et al. on B16 melanoma cells and found to inhibit dopachrome formation.[11]

Dioic Acid

It belongs to the dicarboxylic acid group and acts as agonist to nuclear PPAR, which regulates tyrosinase transcription and melanosome transfer. In an open, comparative, 12 week study on 96 Mexican female patients with melasma dioic acid was found to be an effective and highly tolerated skin product for melasma as compared to 2% HQ.[8]

Linoleic Acid

It is an unsaturated, 18 carbon fatty acid, derived from hydroxylated botanical oils, e.g., safflower. It accelerates tyrosinase degradation and turnover of stratum corneum. Lincomycin is a lincosamide antibiotic, produced by actinomycete, *Streptomyces lincolensis*, which inhibits melanogenesis post-transcriptionally. The efficacy of these drugs is proven in *in vitro* studies.[8]

Umbelliferone or 7-Hydroxycoumarin

It is a phenolic compound found in many plants from the apiaceae (umbelliferae) family, such as carrot and coriander. Umbelliferone absorbs ultraviolet light and also has antioxidant and anti-inflammatory properties.[1]

Box 1: Newer combinations[12]

- Arbutin (deoxyarbutin) and aloesin
- Licorice extract, soy and ascorbic acid (magnesium ascorbyl phosphate)
- Kojic acid, phytic acid, and butylmethoxy dibenzoyl methane
- Azelaic acid 20% and tretinoin 0.05% or 0.1%
- Mequinol 2% and tretinoin 0.01%
- Hydroquinone 2%, kojic acid 2%, and glycolic acid 10%
- Mequinol 2% in combination with 0.01% tretinoin, tetrahexyldecyl ascorbate, glabridin (licorice extract), niacinamide, retinol.

COMBINATION THERAPY

Combination of multiple ingredients in one formulation is preferred in order to synergistically produce pigment lightening by targeting various mechanisms of action mentioned earlier. This increases the efficacy as compared to monotherapy and reduces the risk of adverse effects. Some combinations of skin lightening agents that have been studied in various trials are mentioned in box 1.

CONCLUSION

Melasma has a very complex pathogenesis and further research is required to unravel its intricacies, and thereby develop newer therapies targeting this enigmatic disorder. Although prescription HQ products remain the gold standard, numerous non-hydroquinone, botanical, and other natural ingredients produce significant skin lightening, and newer agents are being discovered by the day. These agents target the key regulatory steps in melanin synthesis and are usually devoid of any significant side effects. Suitable combinations of these agents need to be designed and evaluated on a large-scale clinical trial to provide an appropriate therapeutic tool for this frustrating disorder.

Editor's Note

Of all non-hydroquinone therapies, only kojic acid, azelaic acid, vitamin C, and dioic acid have some evidence in literature regarding their efficacy. More experience is needed with botanicals to substantiate their claims of effectiveness.

REFERENCES

1. Sarkar R, Arora P, Garg VK. Cosmeceuticals for hyperpigmentation: What is available? J Cutan Aesthet Surg. 2013;6:4-11.
2. Draelos ZD. Skin lightening preparations and the hydroquinone controversy. Dermatol Ther. 2007;20:308-13.
3. Alexis AF, Blackcloud P. Natural ingredients for darker skin types: growing options for hyperpigmentation. J Drugs Dermatol. 2013;12:123-7.
4. Lim JT. Treatment of melasma using kojic acid in a gel containing hydroquinone and glycolic acid. Dermatol Surg. 1999;25:282-4.

5. Fitton A, Goa KL. Azelaic acid: a review of its pharmacologicalproperties and therapeutic efficacy in acne and hyperpigmentaryskin disorders. Drugs. 1991;5:780-98.
6. Gillbro JM, Olsson MJ. The melanogenesis and mechanisms of skin-lightening agents—existing and new approaches. Int J Cosmet Sci. 2011;33:210-21.
7. Griffiths CE, Finkel LJ, Ditre CM, et al. Topical tretinoin (retinoic acid) improves melasma. A vehicle-controlled, clinical trial. Br J Dermatol. 1993;129:415-21.
8. Sarkar R, Chugh S, Garg VK. Newer and upcoming therapies for melasma. Indian J Dermatol Venereol Leprol. 2012;78:417-28.
9. Fisk WA, Agbai O, Lev-Tov HA, et al. The use of botanically derived agents for hyperpigmentation: a systematic review. J Am Acad Dermatol. 2014;70:352-65.
10. Zhu W, Gao J. The use of botanical extracts as topical skin-lightening agents for the improvement of skin pigmentation disorders. J Investig Dermatol Symp Proc. 2008;13: 20-4.
11. Tsuji Naito K, Hatani K, Okada K. Modulating effects of a novel skin-lightening agent, alpha-lipoic acid derivative, on melanin production by the formation of DOPA conjugate products. Bioorg Med Chem. 2007;15;1965-75.
12. Kanthraj GR. Skin-lightening agents: New chemical and plant extracts -ongoing search for the holy grail! Indian J Dermatol Venereol Leprol. 2010;76:3-6.

CHAPTER 10

Oral Agents in the Treatment of Melasma

Evangeline B Handog, Maria Suzanne L Datuin

INTRODUCTION

Melasma is an acquired cutaneous hyperpigmentation that predominantly affects sun-exposed areas of the face and neck. It is the most common pigmentary disorder among Asians[1,2] and is more frequently seen in women and in dark-skinned races.[3]

The exact etiopathogenesis is not known but it is believed to be due to the interplay of several factors, namely, exposure to ultraviolet radiation (UVR), hormonal imbalance, genetics, and a reaction to topical cosmetics and skin products.

TRADITIONAL TREATMENT OF MELASMA

To date, no single treatment exists that provides complete and lasting clearance of melasma. Hydroquinone is considered the gold standard among the topical depigmenting agents.[3]

Conversely, hydroquinone has recently been reported to be a cytotoxic and mutagenic compound in mammalian cells and is now banned in several countries. Other agents include kojic acid, azelaic acid, mequinol, and retinoids. Cosmeceutical agents include licorice, arbutin, soy, N-acetyl glucosamine, and niacinamide, among others.

Measures to protect oneself against UVR such as the use of broad-spectrum sunscreens, sun protective clothing, and sun avoidance are all essential in the successful management of melasma.

ORAL AGENTS FOR MELASMA

Recently, systemic agents have been explored as an adjunct in the treatment of melasma and these include tranexamic acid (TA), pycnogenol/procyanidin and *Polypodium leucotomos* (PL).

Tranexamic Acid

Tranexamic acid is perhaps the most studied among the oral agents used to treat melasma. While the exact mechanism by which it exerts its effects in not fully understood, several mechanisms have been proposed.

Tranexamic acid is a synthetic lysine analog that reversibly blocks lysine binding sites on plasminogen molecules. This effectively inhibits plasminogen activator (PA) from converting plasminogen to plasmin. Keratinocytes are known to produce PA and plasminogen molecules are found in epidermal basal cells. Plasmin also has a role in the release of basic fibroblast growth factor, which is a potent growth factor for melanocytes.[4] In animal models, TA has been shown to prevent ultraviolet light-induced pigmentation by preventing the binding of plasminogen to keratinocytes that resulted in a decrease in the tyrosinase activity of melanocytes.[5] Wu et al. reported that research by Zhang et al. demonstrated that TA inhibited melanogenesis by interfering with the catalytic reaction of tyrosinase.[5] Other studies showed that TA is able to decrease α-melanocyte stimulating hormone that stimulates melanin synthesis.[2]

In an open label study involving 74 Chinese females, TA was given at a dose of 250 mg twice daily for 6 months. The patients were advised to wear a sunscreen daily. Two independent physicians assessed patient photographs for a reduction in size and degree of pigmentation. In as early as one month, 82.4% (61/74) of subjects had noticeable improvement which increased to 94.6% (70/74) after two months. At the end of the study, 10.8% (8/74) of subjects had excellent results, 54% (40/74) had good results, 31.1% (23/74) had fair results while 4.1% (3/74) reported poor results. The total improvement rate was seen in 95.9% of the subjects. Side effects were few and mild and included nausea, diarrhea, abdominal pain, hypomenorrhea, skin rashes, alopecia, drowsiness, and hyposexuality. Also notable was that while melasma lesions improved during treatment, non-melasma pigmented lesions such as lentigenes and ephelides remained unchanged. Recurrence in seven subjects occurred in the 6 months follow-up period.[5]

A randomized controlled trial by Karn et al. evaluated the efficacy of TA as an adjunct to topical hydroquinone and sunscreen for melasma in 260 subjects.[3] Group A received TA at a dose of 250 mg twice daily in addition topical treatment and Group B received topical treatment alone for a period of 3 months. The primary outcome measures were a reduction in the Melasma Area Severity Index (MASI) at 8th and 12th weeks and patient satisfaction scores using a four-point scale. Among group A subjects, there was a statistically significant decrease in MASI scores from baseline to 8 weeks ($p < 0.05$) and to 12 weeks ($p < 0.05$). Among group B subjects, decrease in the MASI score was significant at 8 weeks ($p < 0.05$) but not at 12 weeks ($p > 0.05$). Good to excellent results were reported by 82.3% of subjects in group A and 40.8% from group B. Side effects were mild and included oligomenorrhea, belching, abdominal cramps, palpitations, and an urticarial rash with angioedema in one subject. The authors also observed that exogenous ochronosis in two subjects significantly improved with TA.[3]

Pycnogenol/Procyanidin

Pycnogenol, a standardized extract of the bark of the French maritime pine, *Pinus pinaster,* has procyanidin (65–75%) as the main active ingredient.[2] Pycnogenol contains other phenolic compounds such as catechin, epicatechin, caffeic acid, and ferulic acid.[6] It has anti-inflammatory and antioxidant properties, being more potent than vitamins C and E *in vitro*.[1,6,7] It has been demonstrated to protect against UV-induced erythema through mechanisms that inhibit the expression of nuclear factor (NF)-κB.[6] It has high bioavailability and low incidence of side effects.[2]

In an open label trial on 30 Chinese females with melasma, pycnogenol at a dose of 25 mg thrice daily was given for 30 days. Results showed a decrease in pigment intensity ($p < 0.001$) and melasma area ($p < 0.001$) in 80% of the subjects. No side effect was observed, and blood and urine test parameters were within the normal range. In addition to its anti-melasma effects, other symptoms such as fatigue, constipation, body pains, and anxiety also improved.[1]

In a randomized, double bind, placebo-controlled trial, a fixed combination of oral procyanidin plus vitamins A, C, and E was given to 60 Filipino females with bilateral epidermal melasma. The combination containing 24 mg of procyanidin was taken twice daily for 8 weeks and was compared to placebo using melanin index (MI) scores and MASI score analysis. Fifty-six subjects completed the study, with a reduction in MASI scores in both placebo and treatment groups ($p = 0.001$) and a significant reduction between the two groups ($p < 0.0001$). The MI of the right and left malar regions were also significantly reduced at weeks 4 and 8 ($p < 0.0001$). No serious adverse events were reported in the study, however, one subject reported a metallic taste after ingestion of the study drug.[7]

Polypodium leucotomos

Polypodium leucotomos (PL) is a tropical species of fern, whose extract contains various compounds that possess antioxidant and photoprotective properties. It is able to maintain the structural integrity of the extracellular matrix that is usually damaged through UV-induced expression of matrix metalloproteinases.[8]

A review by Nestor et al. quoted a randomized, placebo controlled trial, which evaluated oral PL in 21 females (18–50 years) with epidermal melasma. *Polypodium leucotomos* was given twice daily (dose not stated) for a duration of 12 weeks in addition to daily use of a sunscreen. Outcome measures included change in the Melasma Quality of Life scale (MelasQOL), MASI score, clinical evaluation by the study investigator, and photographic evaluation by an independent, blinded investigator. At the end of the study, subjects who received PL had significantly decreased mean MASI scores ($p < 0.05$) which was not observed in the placebo group. Photographic evaluation revealed 60% improvement in the PL group and 14% improvement in the placebo group. Similarly, patient self-evaluation revealed 63% improvement for the PL group and 17% for the placebo group. In addition, 17% of subjects in the placebo group reported worsening of melasma, as opposed to none in the PL group.[8]

However, an unfavorable result was seen in another study. In a randomized, double-blinded, placebo controlled trial, oral PL was given as an adjunct to sunscreen in the treatment of melasma. Forty Hispanic women with moderate to severe melasma (MI of 30 more) were randomized to receive either 240 mg of PL or placebo three times a day for 12 weeks.

The primary outcome measure was a change in the MI from baseline to 6 weeks and to 12 weeks. Secondary outcome measures were change in the

MASI score and the MelasQOL. Only 33 subjects completed the study. Both treatment and placebo groups had significant decreases in the MI from baseline to 12 weeks, with 28.8% improvement in the treatment group and 13.8% in the placebo group. However, the difference between the two groups was not statistically significant ($p = 0.14$). The intergroup MASI score was not statistically significant ($p = 0.62$) and the MelasQOL showed minimal change in either group. The authors concluded that PL was well tolerated but not significantly better than placebo in the treatment of melasma.[9]

CONCLUSION

While topical therapy and photoprotection are the mainstays in the treatment of melasma, these oral agents hold great promise, either as primary or as adjunctive therapies. Oral agents have the advantage of convenience of use, lack of local cutaneous irritation and possibly better compliance. More randomized controlled trials with larger sample sizes are needed in order to establish their efficacy and safety, as well as to determine the most optimal dosing with the least adverse effects.

Editor's Note

Oral agents, especially tranexamic acid need to be assessed alone and with combination therapy for future use in melasma. Oral agents can well be the third line therapy for melasma.

REFERENCES

1. Ni Z, Mu Y, Gulati O. Treatment of melasma with Pycnogenol. Phytother Res. 2002;16(6): 567-71.
2. Sarkar R, Chugh S, Garg VK. Newer and upcoming therapies for melasma. Indian J Dermatol Venereol Leprol. 2012;78:417-28.
3. Karn D, Kc S, Amatya A, Razouria EA, Timalsina M. Oral tranexamic acid for the treatment of melasma. Kathmandu Univ Med J (KUMJ). 2012;10:40-3.
4. Tse TW, Hui E. Tranexamic acid: an important adjuvant in the treatment of melasma. J Cosmet Dermatol. 2013;12:57-66.
5. Wu S, Shi H, Wu H, Yan S, Guo J, Sun Y, et al. Treatment of melasma with oral administration of tranexamic acid. Aesthetic Plast Surg. 2012;36:964-70.
6. Konda S, Geria AN, Halder RM. New horizons in treating disorders of hyperpigmentation in skin of color. Semin Cutan Med Surg. 2012;31:133-9.
7. Handog EB, Galang DA, de Leon Godinez MA, Chan GP. A randomized, double-blind, placebo-controlled trial of oral procyanidin with vitamins A, C, E for melasma among Filipino women. Int J Dermatol. 2009;48:896-901.
8. Nestor M, Bucay V, Callender V, Cohen J, Sadick N, Wadorf H. Polypodium leucotomos as an adjunct treatment of pigmentary disorders. J Clin Aesthet Dermatol. 2014;7:13-7.
9. Ahmed AM, Lopez I, Perese F, Vasquez R, Hynan LS, Chong B, et al. A randomized, double-blinded, placebo-controlled trial of oral Polypodium leucotomos extract as an adjunct to sunscreen in the treatment of melasma. JAMA Dermatol. 2013;149:981-3.

CHAPTER 11

Chemical Peels for Melasma

Shehnaz Z Arsiwala

INTRODUCTION

Melasma is a chronic acquired hypermelanosis of persistent nature and resistant to therapies with a tendency to recur. No single therapeutic modality is sufficient to achieve total clearance of pigmentation in melasma and maintenance of response is a true challenge. Therefore, therapies need to be combined to optimize the outcome.

Current melasma therapies include:

- Topical therapies
- Oral therapies
- Interventional therapies.

A framework of sequencing therapies constitutes melasma treatment with topical therapies forming the mainstay of the treatment. The primary approach constitutes usage of topical therapies in single, dual, or triple combinations with or without hydroquinone (HQ) along with a broad spectrum sunscreen. The interventions, when sought have to be adjunctive to topical therapies. The practical considerations while executing interventions in melasma are highlighted in box 1.

INTERVENTIONAL THERAPIES

The interventional and procedural based therapies in melasma:

- Chemical peels
- Lasers and lights

Box 1: Practical considerations for interventions in melasma

- Never as first-line therapy
- Always adjuvant to topical therapies
- Introduced for unresponsive or recalcitrant cases
- Recurrences are common and multiple sequential treatments in combinations are required
- Optimum clearance and maintaining remission is difficult

This chapter deals with practical and evidence-based considerations for chemical peeling in melasma.

CONCEPT OF PEELS IN MELASMA

Chemical peels achieve tissue replacement by destruction, elimination, and regeneration of epidermis and a part of dermis all through a controlled stage of inflammation. The peeling agent used can cause elimination of epidermal melanin, elimination of the melanin from the keratinocytes as well as melanosomes transfer to the keratinocytes, thus useful for the epidermal pigment component of melasma. While treating Indian skin types, the superficial peels are often used for safety and prevention of postinflammatory hyperpigmentation over medium depth to deep peels. The superficial peels are helpful, but results may be variable and multiple sessions and rotational treatments may be required, also maintenance with topical therapy is mandatory. Medium depth and high strength peels are effective but risk of postinflammatory hyperpigmentation in skin of color, judicious use and excellent priming as well as post peel care are essential. Recurrence in melasma is very common and pigment improvement may be only partial thus limiting applications of peels in dark skin types.

Peels are never used as a primary choice but as a second line and often used for recalcitrant melasma. While the chemical peels may work to a certain extent on epidermal pigment in melasma, the dermal pigment in melasma does not respond well to peels. Chemical peels can be combined with triple combination formula to hasten the efficacy, especially in mixed epidermal and dermal melasma.

Evidence from literature reflects that clearance of melasma is better and faster when chemical peels are combined with topical therapy. The peels studied are α-hydroxyl acid (AHA) peels like glycolic acid (GA), mandelic acid (MA), β-hydroxyl acid (BHA) peels, e.g., salicylic acid (SA) and combination peels like Jessener's and tretinoin peels. Box 2 highlights favorable features for peels in melasma.

Ground Rule for Peels in Melasma

Conducting peels in an Indian skin differs and cannot be followed along the lines of Fitzpatrick skin type I–III. Peels should be conducted on well informed, sun protected compliant patients with realistic expectations. For skin of color with melasma while conducting peels excellent priming ensures adequate suppression of neomelanogenesis.

Box 2: Favorable features for peels in melasma

- Melasma <1 year of duration (early melasma)
- Epidermal component more favorable than dermal component
- Heterogeneous pigment pattern more favorable than homogenous pigment pattern
- Focal melasma yields better results than extensive pan-facial pattern

PEEL CONSIDERATIONS FOR MELASMA

- Choosing right patient
- Adequate priming
- Choosing right peel—formulation and technique.

Choosing the Right Patient

A sun protected patient who has completed at least 3–5 months of topical therapy should be considered for peels. A right candidate is one with predominant epidermal pigment. Thorough counseling regarding peeling as an adjunctive intervention and emphasis on adherence to topical therapy is crucial. A predominant epidermal pigment as reflected by Woods light examination would be a good candidate for peels. Boxes 2 and 3 highlight favorable features and contraindications for peels in melasma.

Priming before Peels in Melasma[1,2]

Choosing a right and specific priming agent is essential. HQ is gold standard for priming before peels. The depigmenting effects of the HQ treatment become evident after 5–7 weeks. Treatment should be continued for at least 3 months. Peels can be added after 6 weeks of HQ which should be stopped 2 weeks before peels and restarted a week after.

Retinoids as priming agents can be used alone or in combination with kojic acid or arbutin or GA. Tretinoin: priming is most commonly used, at least 4 weeks before peel is introduced. Adapalene and tazarotene can also be used for priming. Adapalene has the advantage of less irritation than tazarotene and tretinoin.

Disadvantage of retinoids is stratum corneum thinning with resultant irritation with increased sun sensitivity in some patients. A good emollient should be added while priming with retinoids. Retinoids should be stopped for a week before peels. One must also ensure to defer a peel procedure when patients exhibit retinoid dermatitis and initiated only when the dryness and inflammation settles down.

GA is the most widely used agent for priming. 6–12% GA is a good priming agent for peels in melasma and can be combined with tretinoin or HQ. GA is started at least 6 weeks before peels and stopped a week before and reintroduced after 5–7 days of peels.

Box 3: Contraindications for peels in melasma

- Dermal component prominent
- Prolonged duration of melasma
- Suspicion of ochronosis
- Unrealistic expectations
- Coexisting inflammatory dermatoses
- Poor priming
- Active bacterial/viral infections
- Keloidal tendency

Box 4: Priming combinations

- HQ: 2–4%
- HQ: 2–4%+ GA: 6–12%
- RA: 0.025–0.05%
- RA: 0.025–0.05% + GA: 6–12%
- 20% Azelaic acid
- 20% Azelaic acid + 0.05% RA
- Vitamin C: 10–15%+ HQ: 2–4% + kojic acid: 2–5%
- Triple combination with fluocinolone acetonide or mometasone for a short period of 12 weeks only

HQ, hydroquinone; RA, retinoic acid.

Combination of agents for priming is gaining ground due to synergism and increased efficacy. Box 4 highlights the combinations of priming agents used. Initial triple combination therapy of HQ, tretinoin and steroid forms a comprehensive priming agent for all cases of melasma; however, the limitations of triple combination warrant for judicious use and patient needs to be switched to monotherapy and non-HQ based therapies between peels in interim phase. Priming has to be initiated for 2–4 weeks before peels, and one should stop retinoids 4–7 days before peels and resume them 4–5 days after.

Kojic acid (KA) is more effective in combination with other agents and is used twice a day for 1–2 months. It is started 3 weeks before peels and stopped a week before and reintroduced after 5 days. It has high sensitizing potential. KA is useful in patients who cannot tolerate HQ.

Sun Protection

- Broad spectrum sunscreen with SPF of 15 or above and UVA coverage should be started well in advance
- Sunscreens have a photosensitizing property in certain patients which can be unmasked before the peel is undertaken
- One must choose a newer photo stable sunscreen with a physical block if possible.

Peeling Agents for Melasma

α-Hydroxy Acid Peels

Glycolic acid peels: 30–70% GA peel as weekly sessions conducted for a series of 4–6 sessions are most commonly conducted peels in melasma. See figures 1 A, B, C, D. Peels are timed from 2–7 minutes of contact and terminated, with increasing percentage of GA in subsequent sessions. Neutralization with sodium bicarbonate solution or cold water is necessary. Gel peels can be used for sensitive skin. Liquid peels have better bioavailability. Free acid peels are preferred over gel peels. Various studies in skin of color highlight value of GA peels and emphasize the significance of increased efficacy when 30–40% GA peels are combined with topical therapies like modified Kligman's formula,

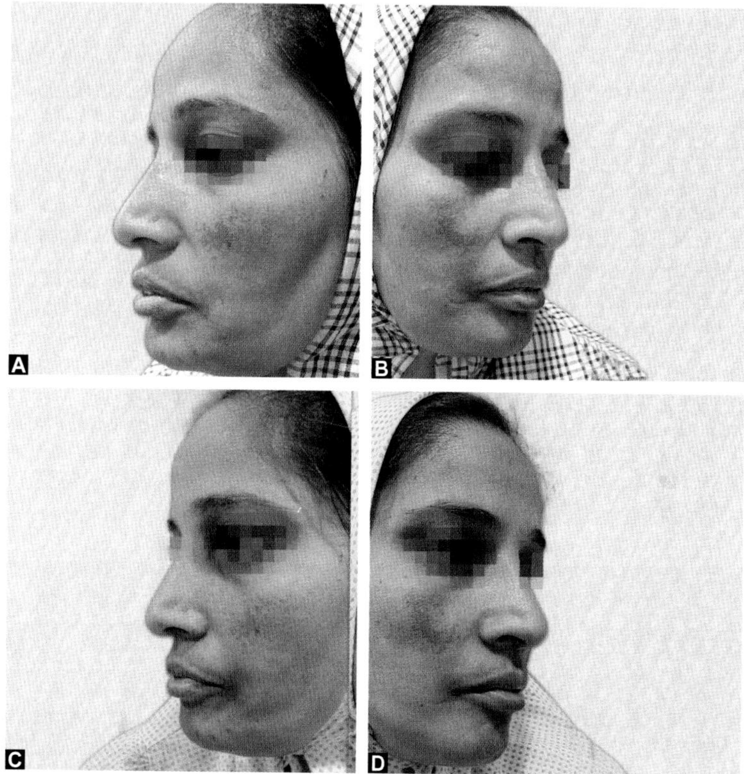

Figure 1: A, Melasma before treatment; **B,** Melasma before; **C,** Melasma improvement after 6 sittings of 35% glycolic acid peels; **D,** Melasma improvement after 6 sittings of 35% glycolic acid peels.

topical 10% GA, topical vitamin C, azelaic acid, and adapalene.[3-7] Some studies reported superior results when GA peel concentration was as high as 50% with topical therapies.[8] Sequencing peels with a triple combination topically has been studied to show a better efficacy in moderate to severe melasma when measured by spectrometry.[7]

Lactic acid (LA) peels are also small molecular weight AHAs and proved beneficial when used as 92% strength at pH 3.5. Double coats of LA are applied for 10 minutes every 3 weeks for epidermal component in melasma and have been compared to Jessener's peel and found to be safe and efficacious.[9]

Mandelic acid at 30–50% applied weekly or biweekly is another agent used for peels in melasma. Advantage over other agents is its anti-inflammatory actions and less erythema and synergistic effect with other peels and lasers.[3]

Phytic acid peels is a GA based slow release peel in combination with mandelic and LA as adjuvants with phytic acid as an antioxidant and peel booster to be applied under occlusion and does not need termination. In melasma, it can be used twice in a month for 4–5 sessions.[3,10]

Tretinoin Peels

Tretinoin peels are useful in melasma where in 5–10% tretinoin is applied as a slow release peel and helps to eliminate epidermal pigment, reduce photo-damage, and improve texture. See figures 2 A, B, C, D. It is beneficial as the patients are already primed with topical tretinoin alone or in triple combination therapy. Tretinoin peels versus GA peels in the treatment of melasma in dark-skinned patients has been studied by Khunger et al. in Indian patients where 1–5%. Tretinoin peel at 1% strength is applied for 4 hours once a week, for 12 weeks and found to be of equal efficacy.[11]

Salicylic Acid Peels

Salicylic peels in 20–30% strength help in elimination of epidermal pigment in well primed patients of melasma. Lipohydroxy acid peel has better keratolytic action and a smoother post peel texture but studies on superior efficacy over SA is lacking. Grimes study (1999) conducted five SA peels 20% and 30% pretreated with HQ 4% resulted in moderate to significant improvement in 4 out of 6 patients of dark skin with melasma. Hyperpigmentation was observed more in patients who were on non-HQ priming agents.[12,13]

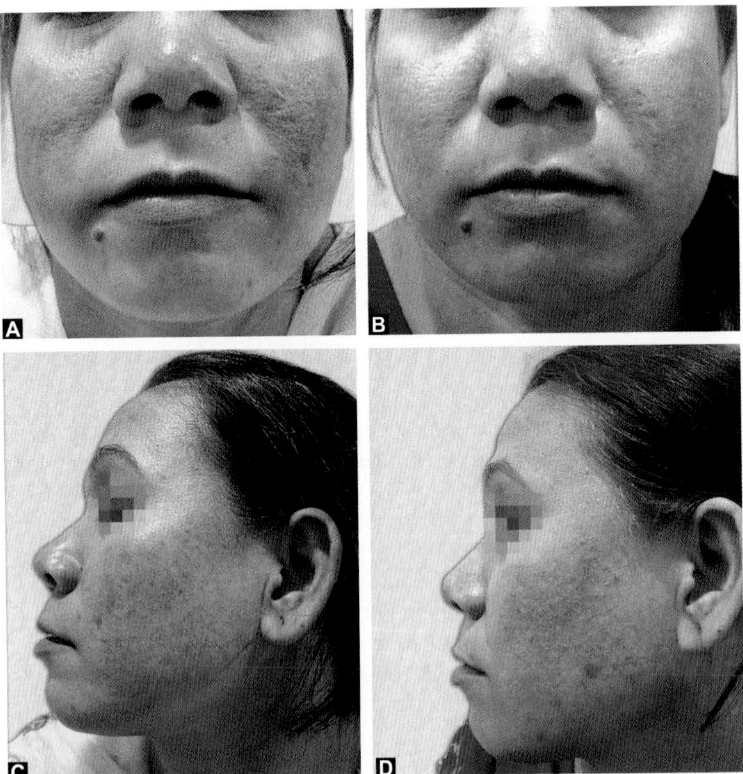

Figure 2: A, Melasma before treatment; **B,** Melasma after yellow peels; **C,** Melasma before treatment; **D,** Melasma after yellow peels.

Trichloroacetic Acid Peels

Trichloroacetic acid (TCA) peels work on principle of causticity. In lower strength of 15%TCA can be used as a superficial peel and at higher strength it can act as a medium depth peel. The TCA peel can be conducted at monthly interval for about 4 sessions and can be done 1–2 coats on melasma zone and single coat pan facially. It is a self-limiting peel and end-point is frosting. Vigilance for postinflammatory hyperpigmentation is required even with low strength TCA peels in skin of color. Single coat of TCA peel creates a superficial peel. Increasing number of coats can make it medium depth. Frosting here acts as a guide to depth control.

A comparative study of TCA versus GA chemical peels in the treatment of melasma reported that GA peel is associated with fewer side effects than TCA and has the added advantage of facial rejuvenation.[14] Kalla et al. reported degree of response was better with TCA but relapses were more common.[15] Topical ascorbic acid combined with 20% TCA peel in melasma improves the results and helps in maintaining the response to therapy[16] and better when TCA is used along with modified Jessener's peel.[17]

Levels of evidence and strength of recommendations for various peeling agents in ethnic skin by US task force grades GA as A level and lactic, salicylic, TCA, and Jessener's as level B recommendation and level C recommendation for phytic and pyruvic acid peels in improvement of melasma. Evidence-based peels with levels of evidence are listed in box 5.

When evaluating a case for peels in melasma, a physician must consider all the possible peel as well as non-peel options available to improve the condition. Choose the ones with best results and minimal side effects. Consider the need to combine various techniques along with peels, e.g., microdermabrasion, lasers, etc.

Glycolic acid, TCA, Jessener's solution, SA, tretinoin, and KA peels are used. GA 20–50% is useful in dark skin types. Dermal melasma is unresponsive to chemical peeling treatment. Clearance of whatever degree requires maintenance with topical therapy. Post peel care as listed in box 6 needs to be followed rigorously in all cases.

Box 5: Evidence-based peels for melasma

- GA: 10–50% (Level of evidence: C)
- GA: 70% (B)
- TCA: 10–25% (C)
- Jessener's peel:—(SA + LA + resorcinol + ethanol) (C)
- SA: 20–30% (C)
- Retinoic acid peel: 1–5% (C)
- KA: 2–5% (C)
- Pyruvic acid: (50%) (C)
- Combinations
- GA (50%) + KA (10%) (C)
- Retinol peel: 5% (C)

GA, glycolic acid; TCA, trichloroacetic acid; SA, salicylic acid; LA, lactic acid; KA, kojic acid.

Box 6: Post peels care

- Post peel care in melasma
- Ice compresses
- Restrict emollients for 2 days
- Once peeling initiates start emollients if visible dryness
- Sunscreens are a must
- Moisturizers may be required
- Advise mild gentle neutral pH facial cleansers
- Restart lightening agents at 1–2 weeks

CONCLUSION

Though chemical peels are an adjuvant therapy in melasma and never used as a first line therapy, they are a beneficial option for elimination or reduction of epidermal component of melanin and efficacy increases when peels are added to topical therapy. A large number of peeling agents are now emerging as evidence-based option for sequential treatment of melasma with topical therapy and sunprotection. Choosing a right patient with adequate priming, adherence to sunprotection, and topical therapy with peels as interventions forms a backbone to improving melasma in the current scenario.

Editor's Note

Chemical peels work best as adjuvants to topical therapies such as hydroquinone, modified Kligman's regime, azelaic acid, kojic acid, and others. They have more rejuvenating effects than lightening of pigmentation. They are useful modalities in the armamentarium of treatment of melasma but good priming is important for preventing post peel hyperpigmentation. Conventional peels are more efficacious but combination and proprietary peels have fewer side effects.

REFERENCES

1. Resnik BI. The role of priming the skin for peels. In: Rubin MG, editor. Chemical peels. Procedures in cosmetic dermatology.1st ed. New Delhi: Elsevier Inc; 2006. pp. 21-6.
2. Fabbrocini G, De Padova MP, Tosti A. Chemical peels:what's new and what isn't new but still works well. Facial Plast Surg. 2009;25:329-36.
3. Sarkar R, Bansal S, Garg VK. Chemical peels for melasma in dark-skinned patients. J Cutan Aesthet Surg. 2012;5:247-53.
4. Sobhi RM, Sobhi AM. A single-blinded comparative study between the use of glycolic acid 70% peel and the use of topical nanosome vitamin C iontophoresis in the treatment of melasma. J Cosmet Dermatol. 2012;11:65-71.
5. Sarkar R, Kaur C, Bhalla M, Kanwar AJ. The combination of glycolic acid peels with a topical regimen in the treatment of melasma in dark-skinned patients: a comparative study. Dermatol Surg. 2002;28:828-32.
6. Lim JT, Tham SN. Glycolic acid peels in the treatment of melasma among Asian women. Dermatol Surg. 1997;23:177-9.
7. Rendon M. Successful treatment of moderate to severe melasma with triple-combination cream and glycolic acid peels: a pilot study. Cutis. 2008;82:372-8.

8. Erbil H, Sezer E, Tastan B, Arca E, Kurumlu Z. Efficacy and safety of serial glycolic acid peels and a topical regimen in the treatment of recalcitrant melasma. J Dermatol. 2007;34:25-30.
9. Sharquie KE, Al-Tikreety MM, Al-Mashhadani SA. Lactic acid chemical peels as a new therapeutic modality in melasma in comparison to Jessner's solution chemical peels. Dermatol Surg. 2006;32:1429-36.
10. Khunger N, Arsiwala S. Combination and Sequential peels.In: Khunger N (Ed). Step by Step Chemical Peels, 1st Edition.New Delhi: Jaypee Brothers Medical Publishers; 2008. pp. 201-18.
11. Khunger N, Sarkar R, Jain RK. Tretinoin peels versus glycolic acid peels in the treatment of melasma in dark-skinned patients. Dermatol Surg. 2004;30:756-60.
12. Grimes PE. The safety and efficacy of salicylic acid chemical peels in darker racial-ethnic groups. Dermatol Surg. 1999;25:18-22.
13. Kodali S, Guevara IL, Carrigan CR, Daulat S, Blanco G, Boker A, et al. A prospective, randomized, split-face, controlled trial of salicylic acid peels in the treatment of melasma in Latin American women. J Am Acad Dermatol. 2010;63:1030-5.
14. Kumari R, Thappa DM. Comparative study of trichloroacetic acid versus glycolic acid chemical peels in the treatment of melasma. Indian J Dermatol Venereol Leprol. 2010; 76:447.
15. Kalla G, Garg A, Kachhawa D. Chemical peeling—glycolic acid versus trichloroacetic acid in melasma. Indian J Dermatol Venereol Leprol. 2001;67:82-4.
16. Soliman MM, Ramadan SA, Bassiouny DA, Abdelmalek M. Combined trichloroacetic acid peel and topical ascorbic acid versus trichloroacetic acid peel alone in the treatment of melasma: a comparative study. J Cosmet Dermatol. 2007;6:89-94.
17. Safoury OS, Zaki NM, El Nabarawy EA, Farag EA. A study comparing chemical peeling using modified Jessner's solution and 15% trichloroacetic acid versus 15% trichloroacetic acid in the treatment of melasma. Indian J Dermatol. 2009;54:41-5.

CHAPTER 12

Lasers for Melasma

Pooja Arora, Rashmi Sarkar

INTRODUCTION

Lasers have revolutionized the treatment of many dermatological conditions. One of these is the pigmentary disorders. Lasers have been widely used with variable success for the treatment of pigmentary disorders including melasma. However, the efficacy and safety of lasers for melasma is still controversial. In this chapter, we have discussed the various lasers that have been tried in melasma.

OVERVIEW OF LASERS

Laser treatment of pigmented lesions is based on the theory of selective photothermolysis proposed by Anderson and Parrish, which states that when a specific wavelength of energy is delivered in a period of time shorter than the thermal relaxation time (TRT) of the target chromophore, the energy is restricted to the target and causes less damage to the surrounding tissue. Hence, a laser should emit a wavelength that is specific and well absorbed by the particular chromophore being treated. A selective window for targeting melanin lies between 630 nm and 1,100 nm, where there is good skin penetration and preferential absorption of melanin over oxyhemoglobin. Absorption for melanin decreases as the wavelength increases, but a longer wavelength allows deeper skin penetration. Shorter wavelengths (<600 nm) damage pigmented cells with lower energy fluencies, while longer wavelengths (>600 nm) penetrate deeper but need more energy to cause melanosome damage.

Besides wavelength, pigment specificity of lasers also depends on pulse width. With an estimated TRT of 250–1,000 ns, melanosomes require submicrosecond laser pulses (<1 ms) for their selective destruction, but longer pulse durations in the millisecond domain do not appear to cause specific melanosome damage. Various lasers that have been used for melasma include the following:

- *Green light*: Flashlamp-pumped pulsed dye laser (PDL) (510 nm), frequency doubled Q-switched neodymium: yttrium aluminium garnet-532 nm (QS Nd:YAG)
- *Red light*: QS ruby (694 nm), QS alexandrite (755 nm)
- *Near-infrared*: QS Nd:YAG (1,064 nm).

Both lasers and intense pulsed light (IPL) have been used in treatment of melasma. The field of laser surgery has been revolutionized by the introduction of the concept of fractional photothermolysis by Manstein and Anderson. Fractional lasers have been used for the treatment of a variety of pigmented lesions including melasma.

Preoperative Preparation (Box 1)

Box 1: Preoperative preparation

- History: Allergy to topical anesthetic, medical condition, treatment (history of isotretinoin use), history of herpes labialis
- Strict sun avoidance
- Topical depigmenting agents: pre- and post-treatment
- Informed consent
- Pretreatment photographs
- Test spots (for Q-switched lasers)
- Counsel patients accordingly to expect reasonable results
- Appropriate eye protection, eye shields, universal precautions

VARIOUS LASERS IN MELASMA

The recurrent and refractory nature of melasma makes it difficult for treatment. Current treatment strategies include medical treatment (triple combination therapy or modified Kligman's regime, hydroquinone, kojic acid, azelaic acid, and vitamin C), chemical peeling, and laser therapy including IPL.

Q-SWITCHED LASERS

The TRT of melanosomes ranges from 50 ns to 500 ns and absorption spectrum of melanin is broad. Q-switched lasers (QS Nd:YAG, QS ruby, QS alexandrite laser) deliver nanosecond pulse duration, hence they selectively target melanosomes with thermal diffusion.

Q-Switched Nd:YAG

Mechanism of Action

The 1,064 nm QS Nd:YAG is well absorbed by melanin and being a longer wavelength causes minimal damage to epidermis and is not absorbed by hemoglobin. The deeper skin penetration is also helpful to target dermal melanin. Low-dose QS Nd:YAG laser induces sublethal injury to melanosomes causing fragmentation and rupture of melanin granules into the cytoplasm. This effect is highly selective for melanosomes as this wavelength is well absorbed by melanin relative to other structures. There is also subcellular damage to the upper dermal vascular plexus which is one of the pathogenetic factors in melasma.[1] The subthreshold injury to the surrounding dermis stimulates the formation of collagen resulting in brighter and tighter skin.

Efficacy

Q-switched neodymium: Nd:YAG is the most widely used laser for the treatment of melasma (Figures 1 and 2). The fluence used is less than 5 J/cm^2, spot size 6 mm, and frequency of 10 Hz. The number of treatment sessions varies from 5 to 10 at 1-week intervals.

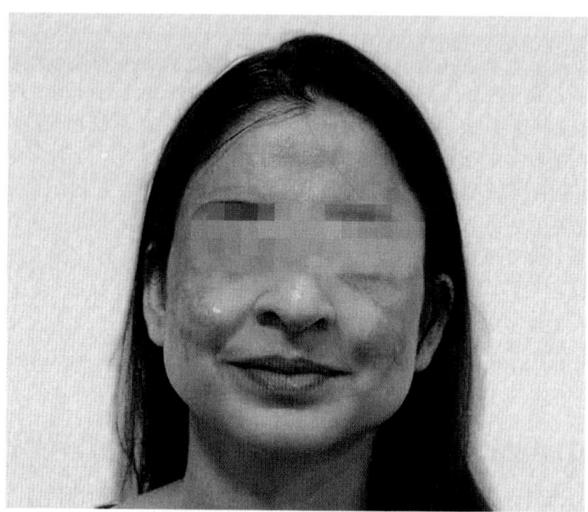

Figure 1: Centrofacial melasma at baseline.
(*Courtesy:* Dr Latika Arya).

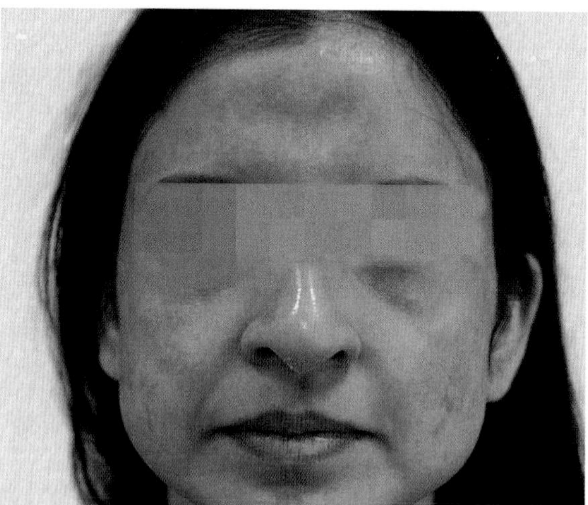

Figure 2: Good improvement in epidermal melasma (50–75%) on Physician Global Assessment scale after 4 sessions of low fluence Q switched Nd:YAG laser, performed every 10 days.
(*Courtesy:* Dr Latika Arya).

A technique called "laser toning" or "laser facial" and has become increasingly popular. It is widely used in Asian countries for skin rejuvenation and melasma. Laser toning involves the use of a large spot size (6–8 mm), low fluence (1.6–3.5 J/cm^2), multiple passed QS 1,064 nm Nd:YAG laser performed every 1–2 weeks for several weeks.[2] While few studies document good efficacy with this technique, several others have found hypopigmentation and depigmentation after a series of laser toning.[2,3] Possible pathogenic mechanisms for this depigmentation could be high fluences causing direct phototoxicity and cellular destruction of melanocyte, subthreshold additive effect of multiple doses, intrinsic unevenness of skin pigmentation, and non-uniform laser energy output.[2] Several other side effects mentioned in the literature include rebound hyperpigmentation, physical urticaria, acneiform eruption, petechiae, and herpes simplex reactivation. Rebound hyperpigmentation could be due to the multiple subthreshold exposures that can stimulate melanogenesis in some areas.

Whitening of fine hair can also occur due to follicular depigmentation. To avoid serious side effects, it is recommended that too many (>6–10) or too frequent (every week) laser sessions with QS Nd:YAG should be avoided. Hypopigmentation should be looked for after every session and further treatments should be stopped.

Q-Switched Ruby Laser

Mechanism of Action

The mechanism is the same as that of QS Nd:YAG laser, that is, it causes highly selective destruction of melanosomes. QS ruby laser (QSRL), being a wavelength of 694 nm, is more selective for melanin than the QS Nd:YAG laser (1,064 nm).

Efficacy

The efficacy of QSRL for melasma is still controversial. So theoretically QSRL is expected to be more effective than QS Nd:YAG for melasma. Tse et al. compared the efficacy and side effect profile of the QSRL and 1,064 nm QS Nd:YAG in the removal of cutaneous pigmented lesions including melasma and found that QSRL provided a slightly better treatment response than the QS Nd:YAG laser.[4] Most patients found QSRL to be more painful during treatment but QS Nd:YAG laser caused more postoperative discomfort. The role of ruby laser is controversial with studies showing conflicting results. More studies are needed to establish its efficacy and safety in melasma.

Erbium:YAG Laser

Mechanism of Action

The erbium:yttrium-aluminium-garnet (Er:YAG) laser emits light with a 2,940 nm wavelength which is highly absorbed by water. Hence, it ablates the skin with minimal thermal damage. The risk of PIH is reduced.

Efficacy

There are very few studies on the use of Er:YAG for melasma. Manaloto et al. treated 10 female patients with refractory melasma using Er:YAG laser at energy levels of 5.1–7.6 J/cm.[5] There was marked improvement of melasma immediately after treatment. However, between 3 weeks and 6 weeks postoperatively, all patients developed PIH that responded well to biweekly glycolic acid peels and topical azelaic acid and sunscreens. The PIH could be due to the inflammatory dermal reaction induced by laser that stimulated the activity of melanocytes in treated skin.

The occurrence of PIH limits the use of this laser for recalcitrant melasma. Moreover, there are hardly any studies documenting its efficacy in melasma.

Pulsed Dye Laser

Mechanism of Action

The use of PDL for the treatment of melasma is based on the theory that skin vascularization plays an important role in the pathogenesis of melasma. Melanocytes express vascular endothelial growth factor receptors 1 and 2 which are involved in the pigmentation process. PDL, which is mainly used for vascular lesions, targets the vascular component in melasma lesions, decreasing the melanocyte stimulation and subsequent relapses.

Efficacy

A study was conducted in 17 patients with melasma who were treated with PDL and TCC.[6] The combination treatment was compared with TCC alone. The laser treatment was started after 1 month of TCC applications. Three sessions were performed at 3 weekly intervals at the following settings: fluence 7–10 J/cm^2 and pulse duration 1.5 ms. The authors found that the combination treatment had greater treatment satisfaction in patients with skin phototypes II and III. PIH was seen in three patients which could be due to pass used for targeting melanin.

Fractional Lasers

Mechanism of Action

Fractional photothermolysis is a new concept in laser therapy in which multiple microscopic zones of thermal damage are created leaving the majority of the skin intact. The latter serves as a reservoir for healing. These multiple columns of thermal damage are called microthermal treatment zones (MTZ) and lead to extrusion of microscopic epidermal necrotic debris (MENDs) that includes pigment in the basal layer. The viable keratinocytes at the wound margins facilitate the migration of MENDs.

There are numerous advantages of fractional laser therapy. The technique does not create an open wound. The stratum corneum is found to be intact after 24 hours of treatment. Hence, the recovery is faster and complications of open wounds such as hyper- or hypopigmentation are avoided. There is less risk of scarring so areas such as neck and chest that are more prone to scarring can be safely treated. Also, greater depths of penetration can be achieved as entire skin surface is not ablated. Hence, dermal melasma can be targeted.

Efficacy

In a randomized controlled trial by Kroon et al.,[7] 20 female patients with moderate to severe melasma were treated with either nonablative fractional laser (performed every 2 weeks for a total of four sessions) or TTT (once daily for 8 weeks). They used a density of 2,000–2,500 MTZ/cm^2 with energy per microbeam of 10 mJ. Improvement was same in both the groups, but treatment satisfaction and recommendation was higher in laser group. Also, recurrence was noted in both the groups. No case of PIH was seen.

Study done by Goldberg et al.[8] has shown a reduced number of melanocytes after fractional laser which implies that this laser delayed pigmentation.

Density used varies from 2,000 MTZ/cm^2 to 2,500 MTZ/cm^2 and energy levels 10–15 mJ/mb. The treatment sessions vary from 2 to 6 at an interval of 1–4 weeks. Levels of improvement vary in different studies.

It can be inferred that topical bleaching agents should be regarded as the gold standard in the therapy of melasma. The treatment is cheap and less painful. Nonablative fractional laser (1,550 nm) is safe and comparable in efficacy and recurrence rate with TTT and should be used only when the latter is ineffective or not tolerated.

Intense Pulse Light

Mechanism of Action

According to Kawada et al., the mechanism of effectiveness of IPL involves absorption of light energy by melanin in keratinocytes and melanocytes leading to epidermal coagulation due to photothermolysis followed by microcrust formation.[9] These crusts containing melanin are shed off hence, the clinical improvement in pigmentation.

Efficacy

Zoccali et al. treated 38 patients with melasma using cut off filters of 550 nm, pulse of 5–10 ms, pulse delay of 10–20 ms, and low fluence 6–14 J/cm^2 and found 80–100% clearance in 47% of patients.[10] The number of sessions used was 3–5 at interval of 40–45 days. No side effects were seen. The laser settings play an important role in the treatment. 500–550 nm filters can be used initially and for epidermal lesions, whereas higher wavelength filters can be used to target deeper melanin in patients with dermal/mixed melasma. The fluence can be modulated in relation to the anatomic sites. Single pulses heat pigment well, but double or triple pulses should be used as they reduce the thermal damage by allowing the epidermis to cool while the target stays warm. The pulse duration used in the studies varied from 3 ms to 5 ms. Average pulse delay used was 10–20 ms. It is important that delay time between pulses should not be below 10 ms as this increases the risk of thermal damage as the targeted tissue cannot reduce its temperature within that time. Average number of sessions used in these studies was 2–5 at an interval of 4–8 weeks. However, more number of sessions is required for maintenance and it decreases the chances of recurrence.

It is a good approach to do a pretest session before starting treatment to assess the efficacy of settings and look for any cutaneous hyper-reactivity.

The studies show that IPL is effective for epidermal melasma. Dermal or mixed or refractory melasma can be targeted with higher fluencies though the risk of PIH should be kept in mind in darker skin. It is a good approach to use low fluences and long delay between pulses in such cases. Also, sun protection and hydroquinone should be used throughout treatment and thereafter.

Patients treated in these studies also had additional benefits of brighter skin color, smoother skin texture, and uniform pigmentation.

Combination of Lasers

Combination of ablative and pigment selective lasers has been tried in melasma. Refractory melasma contains abnormal pigment in both epidermis and dermis. Ablative lasers remove the epidermis (containing excess melanin and abnormal melanocytes). This can be followed by use of Q-switched pigment selective laser that reach deeper lesion in dermis (dermal melanophages) without causing serious side effects.

LASERS IN THE FUTURE

Fractional Erbium-Yag laser has been recently FDA approved for melasma. The Thulium laser and Copper Bromide laser appear promising but have been tried in small number of patients. Results should be reviewed cautiously.

CONCLUSION

Lasers have revolutionized the treatment of dermatological disorders but its place in the management of melasma is still controversial. Various studies documented in this chapter focus on the importance of laser settings to derive maximum efficacy and minimal side effects. Choosing the appropriate laser and the correct settings is vital in the treatment of melasma. Also, topical bleaching agents remain the gold standard of therapy as they are evidence-based, are cheap, and of equal or greater efficacy compared to lasers. So the use of latter should be restricted to cases unresponsive to topical therapy or combination with chemical peels. Appropriate maintenance therapy should be selected to avoid relapse of melasma.

Editor's Note

Lasers at present, do not appear very promising and should be reserved for recalcitrant melasma where modalities such as topical therapies and chemical peels have failed. They thus form the third line of therapy for melasma. Pulsed dye laser, thulium laser, and fractional lasers need to be tried cautiously for future. At best, lasers can be combined with fixed triple combination therapy for maintaining good results.

REFERENCES

1. Kim EH, Kim YC, Lee ES, Kang HY. The vascular characteristics of melasma. J Dermatol Sci. 2007;46:111-6.
2. Chan NP, Ho SG, Shek SY, Yeung CK, Chan HH. A case series of facial depigmentation associated with low fluence Q-switched 1,064 nm Nd:YAG laser for skin rejuvenation and melasma. Lasers Surg Med. 2010;42:712-9.
3. Kim MJ, Kim JS, Cho SB. Punctate leucoderma after melasma treatment using 1064-nm Q-switched Nd:YAG laser with low pulse energy. J Eur Acad Dermatol Venereol. 2009; 23:960-2.
4. Tse Y, Levine VJ, Mcclain SA, Ashinoff R. The removal of cutaneous pigmented lesions with the Q-switched ruby laser and the Q-switched neodymium:yttrium-aluminum-garnet laser: A comparative study. J Dermatol Surg Oncol. 1994;20:795-800.
5. Manaloto RM, Alster TS. Erbium:YAG laser resurfacing for refractory melasma. Dermatol Surg. 1999;25:121-3.
6. Passeron T, Fontas E, Kang HY, Bahadoran P, Lacour JP, Ortonne JP. Melasma treatment with pulsed-dye laser and triple combination cream: A prospective, randomized, single-blind, split-face study. Arch Dermatol. 2011;147:1106-8.
7. Kroon MW, Wind BS, Beek JF, van der Veen JP, Nieuweboer-Krobotová L, Bos JD, et al. Nonablative 1550-nm fractional laser therapy versus triple topical therapy for the treatment of melasma.J Am Acad Dermatol. 2011;64:516-23.
8. Goldberg DJ, Berlin AL, Phelps R. Histologic and ultrastructural analysis of melasma after fractional resurfacing. Lasers Surg Med. 2008;40:134-8.
9. KawadaA, Asai M, Kameyama H, Sangen Y, Aragane Y, Tezuka T, et al. Videomicroscopic and histopathological investigation of intense pulsed light for solar lentigines. J Dermatol Sci. 2002;29:91-6.
10. Zoccali G, Piccolo D, Allegra P, Giuliani M. Melasma treated with intense pulsed light. Aesthetic Plast Surg. 2010;34:486-93.

CHAPTER 13

Melasma and Quality of Life

Shilpa Garg, Rashmi Sarkar, Amit G Pandya

INTRODUCTION

Quality of life (QOL) includes all the factors that have an impact on an individual's life. Health related quality of life (HRQOL) measures the physical, social, and psychological well-being of an individual and evaluates the burden of disease on daily life. Melasma negatively affects the HRQOL of an individual due to its location on the face and disfiguring skin discoloration that it causes. It has been shown to undermine the physical, emotional, psychological, and social functioning of an affected individual. It causes a multitude of psychological problems, including distress, and embarrassment, negative fear of evaluation, loneliness, social isolation, feelings of embarrassment, depression, and anxiety. Since Indian women are more prone to develop melasma due to their dark complexion and exposure to intense ultraviolet radiation, it is essential to measure the impact of melasma on their QOL and also the effect of any treatment on QOL.

ADVANTAGES OF MEASURING QOL

- *Clinical*: In guiding treatment decisions by evaluating the overall effect of skin disease on the patient and to monitor progress after treatment
- *Research*: To demonstrate that a treatment improves both clinical and psychological effects of a disease
- *Audit*: Quality of life is used as a criterion to judge the effectiveness of dermatology services based on patient satisfaction with disease management
- *Political and financial*: Since most skin diseases are not life threatening, they are often below the funding cut-off point for granting agencies. In deciding resource allocation, QOL studies provide evidence of the overall burden of skin disease and impact on patients, helping to compare these diseases to non-dermatological diseases.

HRQOL INSTRUMENTS

Instruments to measure HRQOL are questionnaire based. There are general health questionnaires, dermatology-specific questionnaires, and disease-specific questionnaires. Dermatology-specific instruments measure the impact of skin disease on the patient's QOL whereas disease-specific questionnaires measures the impact of diseases such as melasma on patients. The general health questionnaires are not widely used in dermatology.

- *Dermatology-specific questionnaires*: There are many dermatology-specific questionnaires. The two most commonly used HRQOL instruments are the dermatology life quality index (DLQI) and Skindex. Others include instrument proposed by Whitmore (21 questions assessing impact of skin disease on QOL), the American Medical Association (evaluating permanent skin impairment), Robinson (measuring disability in dermatology), the "leisure questionnaire" (evaluating impact of skin disorders on social activities), the impact of skin disease scale (IMPACT, evaluating the psychiatric morbidity in skin disorders), and the Bother Assessment in Skin Conditions Scale (BASC, evaluating how much patients are bothered by their skin condition using a horizontal visual analog scale).
    - *Dermatology life quality index*: The DLQI is a validated questionnaire that was developed by Finlay and Khan.[1] It contains 10 items which cover various aspects of an individual's life such as feelings, symptoms, daily activity, work, leisure, personal relationships, and treatment. The response of the patient is graded on a four-point scale ranging from "very much" to "not at all". The score of each item is added to give a total score ranging from "0" which represents "no effect" to "30" which represents "highest impairment to QOL". The questionnaire has been translated into various languages. Pichardo et al.[2] used the Mexican Spanish version of the DLQI and found that the mean DLQI score in 25 Latino poultry worker males affected by melasma was 7.5 as compared to 2.8 in men without melasma, the difference being statistically significant.
    - *Skindex*: This questionnaire was formulated by Chren et al.[3] It is a self-administered instrument which has 61 items consisting of two physical and three major psychosocial dimensions. The items include fear, anger, depression, embarrassment, social effects, physical discomfort, and physical limitations. Each of these items is graded on the scale ranging from 0 (no effect) to 4 (maximum effect). This instrument falls short in assessing the emotional well being of the patient and focuses primarily on evaluating the impairment and disability in the physical functioning of an individual.
    - *Skindex-16*: Skindex was condensed to Skindex-29 which was further modified to a brief, single-page Skindex-16 (Table 1).[4] It has superior ability to distinguish between patients with different QOL effects and focuses on how much patients are bothered by the diseases rather than the frequency of diseases. Hence, it is a better tool to assess the patient's handicap from a disease. Balkrishnan et al.[5] in their pilot study of 50 women found that the mean Skindex-16 in women with melasma was 55.8, which reflects the significant impact that melasma has on HRQOL. They also found that psychosocial factors were the predominant contributors to the increased HRQOL burden of melasma.

All these HRQOL instruments measure the impact that various skin diseases have on QOL, including melasma. However, they lack the sensitivity for

Table 1: Items of Skindex-16

During the past week, how often have you been bothered by:		
S. No.	**Items**	**Scale**
1.	Your skin condition itching	sx
2.	Your skin condition burning or stinging	sx
3.	Your skin condition hurting	sx
4.	Your skin condition being irritated	sx
5.	The persistence/reoccurrence of your skin condition	em
6.	Worry about your skin condition (For example: that it will spread, get worse, scar, be unpredictable, etc.)	em
7.	The appearance of your skin condition	em
8.	Frustration about your skin condition	em
9.	Embarrassment about your skin condition	em
10.	Being annoyed about your skin condition	em
11.	Feeling depressed about your skin condition	em
12.	The effects of your skin condition on your interactions with others (For example: interactions with family, friends, close relationships, etc.)	fn
13.	The effects of your skin condition on your desire to be with people	fn
14.	Your skin condition making it hard to show affection	fn
15.	The effects of your skin condition on your daily activities	fn
16.	Your skin condition making it hard to work or do what you enjoy	fn

sx, symptoms; em, emotion; fn, functioning.

Note: Response choices for all items are a continuous bipolar scale with seven boxes anchored by the words "Never Bothered" and "Always Bothered" at the ends.

measuring the effect that pigmentary disorders have on QOL. The DLQI and Skindex measure the burden of the disease by giving equal weight to physical and psychological distress caused by skin diseases. But melasma has a far greater impact on the psychosocial well being of an individual compared to physical aspects,hence a specific scale is required to measure HRQOL in patients with melasma.

- *Disease-specific HRQOL instruments*: Disease-specific questionnaires are more accurate in the assessment of patient with a particular skin disease.
    - *Melasma Quality of Life Scale (MELASQOL)*: This instrument which was devised by Balkrishnan et al.[5] specifically emphasizes the HRQOL issues which are specific to melasma. It evaluates 10 items which primarily focus on the emotional and psychosocial aspects of melasma and ignores the physical symptoms. In the questionnaire, seven items are taken from the Skindex-16 and three items are taken from a skin discoloration questionnaire. The 10 chosen items showed highest correlation with both the Skindex-16 and skin discoloration questionnaire. Each of the items is scored using a Likert scale ranging between 1 (not bothered at all) and 7 (bothered all the time). The MELASQOL score ranges from 7 to 70, with a higher score indicating worse QOL. The various domains of the scale are shown in table 2.

Table 2: Melasma Quality of Life Scale[5]

1.	The appearance of your skin condition
2.	Frustration about your skin condition
3.	Embarrassment about your skin condition
4.	Feeling depressed about your skin condition
5.	The effects of your skin condition on your interaction with other people (e.g., interaction with family, friends, close relationship, etc.)
6.	The effects of your condition on your desire to be with people
7.	Your skin condition making it hard to show affection
8.	Skin discoloration making you feel unattractive to others
9.	Skin discoloration making you feel less vital or productive
10.	Skin discoloration affecting your sense of freedom

Note: Each of these 10 points is graded by the patient on a Likert scale of 1 (not bothered at all) to 7 (bothered all the time).

This instrument which was first compiled in English language has now been translated and validated in various languages, including Spanish, French, Brazilian Portuguese, Persian, and Turkish.

The studies on MELASQOL conducted across various regions in different languages (Table 3) reveal that melasma has significant impact on the QOL as depicted by high mean MELASQOL scores.[5-7,10] Melasma seems to affect various domains of QOL like social life, recreation and leisure, emotional well-being, money matters, physical health, and family relationships. Also the severity of melasma assessed clinically by melasma area severity index (MASI) score does not correlate with the QOL of the affected patients in most of the studies.[5-7] This indicates that the therapeutic decisions cannot be solely based on the clinical findings and must incorporate the psychological impact of the disease on the patient. This also emphasizes the need for a melasma-specific questionnaire like MELASQOL in order to assess the psychosocial aspects of melasma.

A Brazilian Portuguese translation of MELASQOL (MELASQOL-BP)[11] showed a significant improvement in the MELASQOL score from 44.4 to 24.3 after treatment with triple combination cream containing hydroquinone 4%, tretinoin 0.05%, and fluocinolone acetonide 0.01%. In another study,[12] participants reported improvement in HRQOL after treatment with the same cream. Hence HRQOL appears to be a useful tool to monitor response to therapy.

CONCLUSION

As treating physicians, we must not only evaluate, treat, and monitor the physical findings of melasma, but we should also determine the impact that melasma has on the HRQOL of an individual. This aspect of the disease is also important in choosing therapy, as HRQOL can help guide treatment decisions, compare effectiveness of various treatment options, and monitor the disease after treatment is completed.

Table 3: Melasma Quality of Life Scale in Different Languages

Authors	Language of MELASQOL	Sample size	Mean MELASQOL score	Domains of MELASQOL most affected by melasma	Correlation between the QOL and disease severity
Balkrishnan et al.[5]	English language	102 women	36	Social life, recreation and leisure, emotional well-being	Moderate correlation between the QOL and disease severity (MASI)
Freitag et al.[6]	Brazilian Portuguese version (MELASQOL-BP)	85 women	37.5	Emotional well-being	No correlation between the QOL and MASI score
Dominguez et al.[7]	Spanish language (Sp-MELASQOL)	99 women	42	Social life, emotional well-being, physical health, money matters	Moderate correlation between the QOL and MASI score. (MASI score-10 and MELASQOL score-42)
Misery et al.[8]	French language (MELASQOL-F)	28 women	20.9	Family relationships, social life	—
Dogramaci et al.[9]	Turkish language (MELASQOL-TR)	114 women	29.9	Appearance of the skin, frustration, feeling unattractive to others, having a restricted sense of freedom	Statistically significant correlation between the QOL and MASI score
Aghaei et al.[10]	Persian language	147 patients (144 women and 3 men)	52.83	Social life, recreation and leisure, emotional well-being	Statistically significant correlation between the QOL and MASI score

MELASQOL, melasmaquality of life scale; QOL, quality of life; MASI, melasma area severity index.

Editor's Note

The impact of melasma on health related quality of life and the effect of treatment on melasma quality of life scale would tell us how effective a treatment is for melasma in the future.

REFERENCES

1. Finlay A, Khan G. Dermatology Life Quality Index (DLQI)—a simple practical measure for routine clinical use. Clin Exp Dermatol. 1994;19:210-6.
2. Pichardo R, Vallejos Q, Feldman SR, Schulz MR, Verma A, Quandt SA, et al. The prevalence of melasma and its association with quality of life in adult male Latino migrant workers. Int J Dermatol. 2009;48:22-6.
3. Chren MM, Lasek RJ, Quinn LM et al. Skindex, a quality-of-life measure for patients with skin disease: reliability, validity, and responsiveness. J Invest Dermatol. 1996 ;107:707-13.
4. Chren MM, Lasek RJ, SahayAP,Sands LP. Measurement properties of Skindex-16: a brief quality-of-life measure for patients with skin diseases. J Cutan Med Surg. 2001;5:105-10.
5. Balkrishnan R, McMichael AJ, Camacho FT, Saltzberg F, Housman TS, Grummer S, et al. Development and validation of a health-related quality of life instrument for women with melasma. Br J Dermatol. 2003;149:572-7.
6. Freitag FM, Cestari TF, Leopoldo LR, Paludo P, Boza JC. Effect of melasma on quality of life in a sample of women living in southern Brazil. J Eur Acad Dermatol Venereol. 2008;22:655-62.
7. Dominduez AR, Balkrishnan R, EllzeyAR,Pandya AG. Melasma in Latino patients: cross-culture adaptation and validation of a quality-of-life questionnaire in Spanish language. J Am Acad Dermatol. 2006;55:59-66.
8. Misery L, Schmitt AM, Boussetta S, Rahhali N, Taieb C.. Melasma: measure of the impact on quality of life using the French version of MELASQOL after cross-cultural adaptation. Acta Derm Venereol. 2010;90:331-2.
9. Dogramaci AC, Havlucu DY, InandiT,Balkrishnan R. Validation of a melasma quality of life questionnaire for the Turkish language: the MelasQoL-TR study. J Dermatolg Treat. 2009;20:95-9.
10. Aghaei S, Moradi A, Mazharinia N, Abbasfard Z. The Melasma Quality of Life scale (MELASQOL) in Iranian patients: a reliability and validity study. J Eur Acad Derm Venereol. 2005;19.
11. Cestari TF, Hexsel D, Viegas ML, Azulay L, Hassun K, Almeida AR, et al. Validation of a melasma quality of life questionnaire for Brazilian Portuguese language: the MelasQoL-BP study and improvement of QoL of melasma patients after triple combination therapy. Br J Dermatol. 2006;156:13-20.
12. Balkrishnan R, Kelly AP, McMichael A, Torok H. Improved quality of life with effective treatment of facial melasma. The pigment trial. J Drugs Dermatol. 2004;3:377-81.

CHAPTER 14

Melasma in Men

Rashmi Sarkar, Shilpa Garg

INTRODUCTION

Melasma is an acquired characteristic pattern of light-to-dark brown facial hyperpigmentation involving the sun-exposed areas. It is more commonly seen in women of child-bearing age and in dark-skinned individuals of Hispanic, Asian, and African origin.[1]

EPIDEMIOLOGY

Melasma is more commonly seen in women as compared to men. However, barring few studies, there is a paucity of studies on melasma in men.

In a study by Vazquez et al.[2] from Puerto Rico, South America, men constituted only 10% of the cases of melasma. In contrast to this low incidence of melasma in Caucasian men, melasma is more commonly reported in men of Indian and Hispanic origin. In a study conducted by Pichardo et al.[3] on Latino men with melasma, data was pooled from three population studies. The prevalence of melasma reported from these three studies which included 25 poultry workers, cross-sectional study of 55 farm workers, and longitudinal study of 300 farm workers were 36.0%, 7.4%, and 14.0%, respectively. The prevalence of melasma across all the three studies was found to be 14.5%.

An Indian study by Sarkar et al.[4] in the year 2003 screened 120 patients of melasma and found that 31 (25.83%) of them were men. Out of these 31 male patients, 18 (58.06%) were outdoor workers with 33.33% being policemen, 33.33% security guards, 11.11% construction engineers, and 22.22% labors who worked at construction sites. In another study by Sarkar et al.,[5] 41 (20.5%) men with Fitzpatrick skin type III–V were identified as having melasma amongst 200 patients who were screened. Twenty four (58.5%) men were outdoor workers and 12 (29.3%) men originally belonged to hilly regions of North India. This greater prevalence of melasma in Indian men as compared to Caucasians could be due to their darker complexion as compared to Caucasians, greater sun exposure due to their outdoor occupation, Indian climate with its hot, long, and dry summers and shorter winters and increased cosmetic awareness amongst men.

ETIOLOGY

The etiological factors causing melasma in men are same as those implicated in women except for the hormonal factors (pregnancy, oral contraceptive pills, hormonal therapy and mild ovarian dysfunction[6]) which are considered as one of the most important etiological factors in causing melasma in women and probably do not hold a causative significance in men[1] (Table 1). This may also explain the relatively low incidence of melasma in men as compared to women. Besides the hormonal factors other factors which are common between both men and women in causing melasma are sunlight, genetic factors, cosmetics, thyroid dysfunction, phototoxic, and anti-seizure medications. Certain chronic diseases like nutritional and hepatic disorders and parasitic infestation have been implicated, although there is no clear evidence in their support.

Table 1: Etiological factors and clinical features of melasma in men and women[5]

Characteristics		Men (n = 41)	Women (n = 159)	p value
Aggravating factors	Sunlight	20 (48.8%)	38 (23.9%)	<0.05*
	Use of mustard oil	18 (43.9%)	50 (31.4%)	>0.05*
	Family history	16 (39.0%)	32 (20.1%)	<0.05*
	Chronic illness (post-typhoid period, thyroid disorder, inflammatory bowel disease)	5 (22.2%)	32 (20.1%)	>0.05*
	Phenytoin	3 (7.3%)	2 (1.3%)	NA
	Pregnancy	0	72 (45.3%)	NA
	Oral contraceptives	0	31 (19.4%)	NA
Age	Mean age (years)	33.5	31.5	>0.05**
	Range of age (years)	19–53	20–45	NA
Duration of melasma (years)		0.1–8.0	0.6–7.0	NA
Mean duration of melasma (years)		3.5	3.1	>0.05**
Clinical pattern of melasma	Centrofacial	12 (29.3%)	81 (51.0%)	<0.001***
	Malar	25 (61%)	39 (24.5%)	<0.001***
	Mandibular	4 (9.7%)	39 (24.5%)	<0.001***
Wood light examination	Epidermal	28 (68.3%)	90 (56.6%)	0.85***
	Mixed	9 (22.0%)	44 (27.7%)	0.85***
	Dermal	4 (9.7%)	25 (15.7%)	0.85***
Histopathological examination	Epidermal	10/20 (50%)	25/40 (62.5%)	
	Mixed	9/20 (45%)	12/40 (30%)	
	Dermal	1/20 (5%)	3/40 (7.5%)	

NA, not applicable for significant testing.
*Z-test for testing difference between two different sample proportions
**Independent sample t-test
***χ^2-test of significance; <0.001 highly significant; <0.05 significant.

In most of the studies[2,4,5] on melasma in men (Table 2), exposure to sunlight and family history were identified as the most common etiological factors for causing melasma and there was a statistically significant difference between men and women (Table 1). In women pregnancy (45.3%), sunlight (23.9%) and oral contraceptives (19.4%) were the major aggravating factors (Table 1).

Amongst the cosmetics used by men, Sarkar et al.[5] reported the application of mustard oil in 43.9% of men with melasma which was in concordance with their earlier study.[4] Mustard oil is derived from the seeds of the mustard plant, which belongs to the family *Brassicaceae*. In certain states of India, this oil is used for cooking, body and hair massage, especially by men.[4] Mustard oil is a common photosensitizer in the Indian setup and can lead to facial pigmentation.

Table 2: Characteristics of melasma in men

Author		Sarkar et al.[4]	Sarkar et al.[5]	Vazquez et al.[2]	Sialy et al.[7]
Total number of patients		Men (n = 31)	Men (n = 41)	Men (n = 27)	Men (n = 15)
Aggravating factors	Sunlight	14 (45.16%)	20 (48.8%)	18 (66.6%)	—
	Family history	5 (16.13%)	16 (39.0%)	19 (70.4%)	—
	Drug (Phenytoin)	2 (6.45%)	3 (7.3%)	0	—
	Use of mustard oil		18 (43.9%)	0	
	Cosmetics (soaps, shaving creams, aftershave, perfumes)			25 (92.6%)	
	Chronic illness (post-typhoid period, thyroid disorder, inflammatory bowel disease)	5 (22.2%)			
Age	Range of age (years)	19–43	19–53	25–72	20–40
	Mean (years)	34.5	33.5	38.8	
Duration of melasma		2 months–4 years	1 month–8 years		2 months–1.5 years
Mean duration of melasma (years)		1.4	3.5	8	
Clinical pattern of melasma	Centrofacial	15 (48.39%)	12 (29.3%)	12 (44.1%)	12 (80%)
	Malar	16 (51.61%)	25 (61%)	12 (44.1%)	2 (13.3%)
	Mandibular	0	4 (9.7%)	3 (11.1%)	1 (6.7%)
Wood light examination	Epidermal	15 (48.39%)	28 (68.3%)	18 (66.6%)	
	Mixed	6 (19.35%)	9 (22.0%)	2 (7.4%)	
	Dermal	10 (32.26%)	4 (9.7%)	7 (25.9%)	
Histopathological examination	Epidermal		10/20 (50%)	4/5 (80%)	
	Mixed		9/20 (45%)	1/5 (20%)	
	Dermal		1/20 (5%)	0	

However, more studies are needed to substantiate the role of mustard oil in causing melasma. In the study by Vazquez et al.,[2] use of various cosmetics like soaps, shaving creams, perfumes, and aftershave were identified in 25 (92.6%) men with melasma, although none of the patients attributed the development of melasma with the use of cosmetics.

Amongst the drugs (Table 2), only phenytoin was found as a causative agent in 6.45% and 7.3% men with melasma in the studies by Sarkar et al.[4,5]

Laboratory investigations in the study by Sarkar et al.[5] revealed anemia in 5 (12.2%) men, giardiasis in 2 (4.9%) men, and increased leuteinizing hormone (LH) and low testosterone in 4 (9.7%) men. Similar hormonal profile was reported in another Indian study[7] which compared 15 male patients of melasma with 11 age matched controls and found that the circulating LH was significantly higher and testosterone was markedly low in the melasmic men concluding that male melasma involves subtle testicular resistance. Similarly, presence of subtle ovarian resistance has been reported in women with melasma.[6]

CLINICAL FEATURES

In the first study group comprising of poultry workers in the study by Pichardo et al.[3] on Latino men, the prevalence of melasma was highest (70%) in men older than 31 years and melasma was absent in men aged 18–24 years. In the rest of the two study groups of farm workers, melasma was prevalent across all the age groups, although its prevalence was highest in men older than 31 years. In concordance with this study, both the studies by Sarkar et al.[4,5] reported the mean age of melasma in men to be 33.5[5] years and 34.5[4] years. Of the 41 men with melasma in the study by Sarkar et al.,[5] 21 (51.2%) men were in the age group of 31–40 years, 11 (26.8%) men were between 19–30 years and 9 (22%) men were 41 years and older. However, in contrast to these findings, Vazquez et al.[2] observed a higher average age (38.8 years) of melasma in men.

In the study by Vazquez et al.[2] and Sarkar et al.,[5] the clinical and histological characteristics of melasma in men were same as those for women barring hormonal factors which did not seem to play a significant role in men (Tables 1 and 2). Malar type of melasma was the most common clinical pattern seen in male patients which was observed across all the studies[2,4,5,7] (Table 2) as compared to women in whom the centrofacial pattern was the most common (Table 1). The difference between the clinical pattern of melasma between men and women in the study by Sarkar et al.[5] was found to be statistically significant (Table 1).

Woods lamp examination of melasma revealed the epidermal pattern to be the most common in men across all the studies (Table 2).

In the study by Sarkar et al.,[5] histopathological analysis was done in 20 (48.8%) men with melasma and 40 (25%) women with melasma and the changes were similar in both men and women (Table 1) with the epidermal pattern of pigmentation being the most common. Additional histopathological features seen were solar elastosis in 17 (85%), flattening of rete ridges in 9 (45%) and infiltration by chronic inflammatory cells in 6 (30%) male patients with no evidence of basal layer degeneration. In the study by Sarkar et al.[5] and Vazquez et al.,[2] epidermal type of melasma was the predominant histopathological type seen in men (Table 2). As the epidermal variety of melasma is more amenable to treatment, melasma in men could be more responsive to treatment.

MELASMA AND QUALITY OF LIFE IN MEN

Though melasma is less commonly seen in men as compared to women, nevertheless it can negatively affect the quality of life (QoL) in men. In the study by Pichardo et al.,[3] there was a statistically significant difference in the Dermatology Life Quality Index (DLQI) in men with and without melasma (7.5 vs. 2.8) in the group of poultry workers. However, there was no statistically significant difference in the DLQI between men with and without melasma in the other two groups of farm workers.

TREATMENT

Melasma in men is approached and treated in the same manner as in women. Efforts should be made to identify and remove the etiological factors and to instill sunprotective behavior in the patient. Treatment options include use of sunscreens, depigmenting creams, peels, dermabrasion, and lasers.

CONCLUSION

Melasma is definitely less common in men as compared to women, although its prevalence is found to be high in Indian and Latino men. The clinicohistopathological characteristics of melasma are same in both men and women. It negatively affects the QoL in men as it does in women and since the epidermal type of melasma is the predominant histopathological type seen in men, it could be more responsive to treatment.

Editor's Note

Melasma is more frequent in dark skinned males and those who spend a longer time outdoor in the sun.

REFERENCES

1. Grimes PE. Melasma. Etiologic and therapeutic considerations. Arch Dermatol. 1995;131: 1453-7.
2. Vazquez M, Maldonado H, Benmaman C, Sanchez JL. Melasma in men. A clinical and histologic study. Int J Dermatol. 1988;27:25-7.
3. Pichardo R, Vallejos Q, Feldman SR, Schulz MR, Verma A, Quandt SA, et al. The prevalence of melasma and its association with quality of life in adult male Latino migrant workers. Int J Dermatol. 2009;48:22-6.
4. Sarkar R, Jain RK, Puri P. Melasma in Indian males. Dermatol Surg. 2003;29:204.
5. Sarkar R, Puri P, Jain RK. Melasma in men: a clinical, aetiological and histological study. J Eur Dermatol Venereol. 2010;24:768-72.
6. Perez M, Sanchez JL, Aquilo F. Endocrinologic profile of patients with idiopathic melasma. J Invest Dermatol. 1983;81:543-5.
7. Sialy R, Massan I, Kaur I, Dash RJ. Melasma in men: A hormonal profile. J Dermatol. 2000;27:64-5.

Treatment Algorithm for Melasma

Assess clinically and with Wood's Lamp (wherever possible). Treat any triggering medical factor.

Photoprotection: Broad spectrum sunscreen (Min PA+ + +, with inorganic sunscreens—TiO_2 or ZnO); Physical barrier

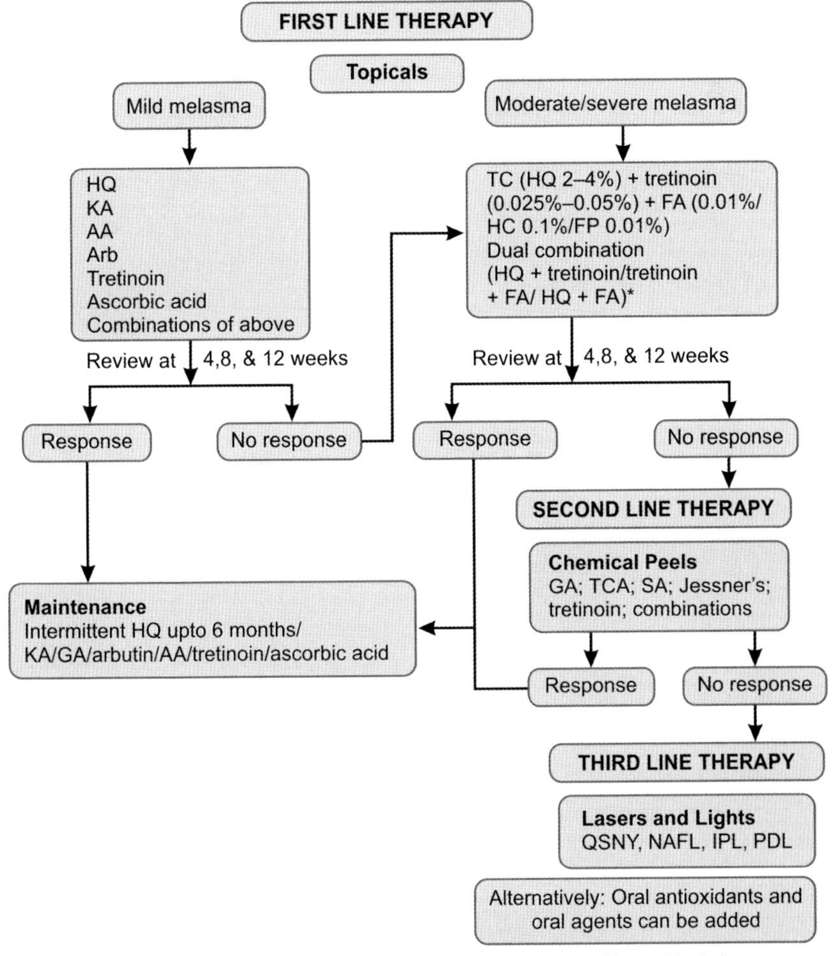

*To stop treatment anytime ochronosis is detected or side effects of topical steroids are detected.

TC, triple combination or modified Kligman's regime; FA, fluocinolone acetonide; FP, fluticasone propionate; HQ, hydroquinone; KA, kojic acid; AA, azelaic acid; Arb, arbutin; GA, glycolic acid; TCA, trichloroacetic acid; SA, salicylic acid; QSNY, Q-switched Nd:YAG laser; NAFL, non-ablative fractional laser; IPL, intense pulse light; PDL, pulsed dye laser.

ACKNOWLEDGEMENT AND REFERENCE

Sarkar R, Ravichandran G, Majid I, Sakhiya J, Godse K, Arya L, Singh M, Sachdev M, Gokhale N, Sarma N, Torsekar RG, Gogoi R, Aurangabadkar S, Rastogi S, Arsiwala S, Sonthalia S, Ghosh S, Shah S, Salim T, Somani VK. Treatment Algorithm for melasma in Indian patients. Consensus meeting of South Asian Pigmentary Disorders Forum (SPF) in association with Pigmentary Disorders Society (PDS), 2014 (Collaborated by Galderma). (Ahead of print).